NewHope

FOR ————————————

People with

Lupus

Other Books in the NEW HOPE Series

New Hope for Couples with Infertility Problems

New Hope for People with Alzheimer's and Their Caregivers

New Hope for People with Bipolar Disorder

New Hope for People with Borderline Personality Disorder

New Hope for People with Depression

New Hope for People with Diabetes

New Hope for People with Fibromyalgia

New Hope for People with Weight Problems

New Hope

FOR

People with
Lupus

Theresa Foy DiGeronimo, M.Ed.

Foreword and Medical Review by
Stephen A. Paget, M.D.

 THREE RIVERS PRESS
NEW YORK

Published by Three Rivers Press, New York.
Member of the Crown Publishing Group, a division of Random House, Inc., New York.
www.crownpublishing.com

THREE RIVERS PRESS and the Tugboat design are trademarks of Random House, Inc.

Originally published by Prima Publishing, Roseville, California, in 2002.

In order to protect their privacy, the names of some individuals cited in this book have been changed.

Interior design by Peri Poloni, Knockout Design
Illustrations by Laurie Baker-McNeile
Medical reviewer photo by Brad Hess

Printed in the United States of America

Library of Congress Cataloging-in-Publication Data
DiGeronimo, Theresa Foy.
   New hope for people with lupus : your friendly, authoritative guide to the latest in traditional and complementary solutions / Theresa Foy DiGeronimo.
      p. cm.—(New hope)
   Includes index.
   1. Systemic lupus erythematosus—Popular works. I. Title. II. Series.
RC924.5.L85 D544   2002
616.7'7—dc21   2001055456

ISBN 0-7615-2097-X

10 9 8 7 6 5

First Edition

To all those who have shared
their stories of lupus in the
hope of helping others.

Contents

Foreword by Stephen A. Paget, M.D.   *ix*

Acknowledgments   *xiii*

1. What Is Lupus?   1

2. Diagnosis   39

3. Medical Treatment   65

4. Complementary and Alternative Therapies   99

5. Nutrition and Exercise   131

6. The Mind-Body Relationship   157

7. Living Well with Lupus   189

8. The Future   233

Appendix: Resources   *253*

Notes   *257*

Glossary   *267*

Index   *273*

Foreword

AFTER CARING FOR people with lupus for nearly 30 years
and being part of academic institutions searching for its causes
and cures, such as Johns Hopkins, the National Institutes of Health,
and the Hospital for Special Surgery, there are a few things that I can
say for sure about the internal terrorist called lupus. There is not only
hope, but also assurance that we will overcome this illness, just as we
did polio, tuberculosis, and rheumatic fever. It is the most complex of
disorders clinically, immunologically, and therapeutically, but it is not
invincible and its secrets are there to be uncovered—and they will be.
We have come a very long way and, although we still have a way to
go, people with lupus should appreciate that while they are fighting
the good fight against lupus in partnerships with their doctors, we are
chipping away rapidly at its immunological core. While we work to
unmask this unpredictable, waxing and waning, invisible, and stealthy
illness, people with lupus, their families, and their doctors should work
together to determine the best treatment approach for each individual.
Until those major breakthroughs are announced, we must all dedicate
our energies to making the lives of people with lupus the best and
most fulfilling they can be by spreading the word about diagnosis and
treatment to both patients and doctors. Our goal is nothing less than
making sure that when it is present, lupus is immediately diagnosed
and appropriately treated. Suffering for years without a diagnosis or

being treated with medications without concern for their cumulative side effects is unacceptable in this age of modern medicine.

Thank goodness there is finally a comprehensive, up-to-date, and accurate resource for people with lupus. *New Hope for People with Lupus* brings to you the most modern concepts in lupus care and addresses, "in one fell swoop," all of the important, scary, hard-to-understand aspects of lupus in a wonderfully readable and understandable form. It not only gives hope because it describes the many advances in our knowledge about and treatment of lupus, but it also enables you to be an informed consumer of medical care, appreciate the complexities of this systemic autoimmune disorder, and approach the disease "head on." Use it as a friend, a guide, a consultant, and show it to your family, your friends, and your doctor. Knowledge gained from this book will move you from a state of fear, misunderstanding, insecurity, and dread to one that can, in close partnership with caring and knowledgeable physicians, improve your quality of life. It does so by helping you to maintain a well-balanced approach to this chronic illness, which in turn enables you to live a longer and happier life.

Lupus is a complex disorder to physicians and researchers in the field, so it is no wonder that it is so misunderstood by patients. It is also an invisible disorder, often missed by physicians for many years because it masquerades as many other illnesses. The patient is often diagnosed as having an infection, chronic fatigue syndrome, fibromyalgia, or even a psychological problem. This book allows you to become a central player in the collaborative diagnostic and therapeutic process that is what medical care is all about. It turns complex into understandable, fear into control, vagueness into solidity and a dark, ill-defined future into a more predictable one. With excellent and beautifully handled chapters on diagnosis, treatment, and other rarely addressed issues such as complementary care, nutrition, maintaining a job, sex, and depression related to having a chronic disorder, *New Hope for People with Lupus* allows you to take charge and move on with your life. It gives hope because there is hope, particularly after absorbing the pearls in this new partner in your medical care.

> —Stephen A. Paget, M.D.
> Physician-in-Chief and Chairman of the Division
> of Rheumatology at Hospital for Special Surgery,
> New York; and the Joseph P. Routh Professor of
> Medicine and Rheumatic Disease at Weill Medical
> College of Cornell University

Acknowledgments

A DEBT OF gratitude and thanks is due to all the professionals who willingly shared their expertise to make this book as accurate and up-to-date as possible: Amy C. Brown, Ph.D., R.D., University of Hawaii, Honolulu; Michael Carroll, M.D., Center for Blood Research, Harvard Medical Center, Boston; Penny Cowan, American Chronic Pain Association, Rocklin, California; Katherine Fox, Davis, California; Anthony Gaspari, M.D., University of Maryland School of Medicine, Baltimore; Michael Gross, M.D., Fair Lawn, New Jersey; Helen Grusd, Ph.D., Los Angeles; Robert Hayden, Evanston, Illinois; Robert S. Katz, M.D., Presbyterian St. Lukes Medical Center, Chicago; Karen Kaufman, Fiskdale, Massachusettes; Robert P. Kimberly, M.D., University of Alabama, Birmingham; Celina Klee, The Upledger Institute, Palm Beach Gardens, Florida; Neil Kurtzman, M.D., Texas Tech University Health Sciences Center, Lubbock; Jimmy Lawrence, M.D., Nemours Clinic, Pensacola, Florida; Matthew Linnik, Ph.D., La Jolla Pharmaceutical, San Diego, California; Michael D. Lockshin, M.D., Hospital for Special Surgery, New York City; Kate Lorig, R.N., Dr.PH., Stanford Patient Education Research Center, Palo Alto, California; Edward J. Madara, M.S., American Self-Help Clearinghouse, Cedar Knolls, New Jersey; LindaSusan Markus, M.D., Wyckoff, New Jersey; Mary-Jo Myers, Pennsylvania School of Muscle Therapy, Oaks, Pennsylvania; Katina Rodis, Ph.D., Concord, Massachusettes; Gloria Spadaro, Lupus Foundation, Elmwood Park, New

Jersey; Margrey Thompson, TheraCare Rehabilitation Companies, Murfreesboro, Tennessee; Ann Traynor, M.D., Northwestern University, Chicago; Ronald F. Van Vollenhoven, M.D., Ph.D., Karolinska Hospital, Stockholm, Sweden; Daniel Wallace, M.D., Wallace Rheumatic Center, Los Angeles; and John Yee, M.D., Veritas Medicine, Cambridge, Massachusettes.

Special thanks to those who shared their personal experiences with lupus: Roxanne Black, Virginia Carpenter, Joanne Forshaw, Kim Jenkins, Donna Lombardo, Mary McDonough, Tiffany Nadeau, Orlando C. Ojeda, Stefanie Oppenheim, Deidre Paknad, Eugene M. Trabosh, Gwendolyn Young, and Sheri Ziemann.

I would also like to thank my helpful and competent editors, Jamie Miller and Marjorie Lery. And I am indebted to Dr. Stephen A. Paget for his thoughtful and competent review of this manuscript.

New Hope

FOR ——————————————————

People with

Lupus

CHAPTER 1

What Is Lupus?

IF YOU OR someone you love has lupus, you probably have a lot of questions—and not many answers. This is a complex and confusing illness that is hard to neatly define and understand. Its symptoms and course vary from one person to the next, and the prognosis depends on many individual factors. So the answer to the simple question, "What's lupus?" is really not so simple.

Literature from the Lupus Foundation of America (LFA) tells us: "Lupus is a chronic inflammatory disease that can affect various parts of the body, especially the skin, joints, blood, and kidneys."[1] But you know that this doesn't explain the half of it. According to Michael D. Lockshin, M.D., director of the Barbara Volcker Center for Women and Rheumatic Disease at Cornell University Medical School in New York, lupus can be "serious or trivial, disfiguring or unnoticeable, painful or painless, life threatening or of little consequence."[2] Certainly, it is not a simple or ordinary disease.

Still, there is good news and reason for hope. Medical experts today know much more about this disease than they did even 10 years ago. People with lupus are starting to get the recognition and treatment they need and deserve. And researchers are now studying the genetic component that may unlock the mysteries of this disease. It is through the continued growth of knowledge and understanding that lupus will be best diagnosed, treated, and managed. This chapter explains what is known at this time about the types, cause, history, symptoms, triggers, prevalence, and prognosis of this complicated disease, so you can better understand what's happening to your body and take an active part in managing your own health.

FOUR TYPES OF LUPUS

The word *lupus* itself is hard to explain. In the thirteenth century, it was thought that the facial rash that sometimes accompanies lupus looked somewhat like the bite mark of a wolf. So, the disease was named lupus, the Latin word for "wolf," although this name has nothing to do with the symptoms or cause of the illness. Medical experts have learned much about this disease since it was named so long ago. Researchers have identified four different types of this noncontagious disease: systemic, drug-induced, discoid, and neonatal.

> *People with lupus are starting to get the recognition and treatment they need and deserve. And researchers are now studying the genetic component that may unlock the mysteries of this disease.*

Systemic Lupus

Systemic lupus erythematosus (SLE or LE) is the form of the disease most often described by the general term *lupus. Systemic* means "all over," and *erythematosus* means "red." This form of lupus is also sometimes called *idiopathic lupus*, meaning "cause unknown." It can affect almost any organ or system of the body.

SLE that presents with many of the common symptoms, but does not affect internal organs is called non-organ threatening disease. Daniel J. Wallace, M.D., clinical professor of medicine at UCLA, who has treated over a thousand lupus patients, tells us that people with this form of lupus (which affects approximately 35 percent of lupus patients and can range from mild to moderate disease) have a normal life expectancy, and it is uncommon for them to develop disease in the major organs after the first five years of having SLE.

SLE that does involve major organs such as the heart, lungs, kidneys, or brain or that causes serious blood abnormalities is called *organ-threatening disease*. It can become life threatening if not properly treated and monitored. Approximately 35 percent of people with lupus fall into this category.[3]

Drug-Induced Lupus

Some people (approximately 10 percent of those with lupus) develop the symptoms of lupus for the first time after taking certain prescription drugs.[4] Although more than 70 agents have been implicated in causing drug-induced lupus erythematosus (DILE), the top three drugs known to cause the symptoms of lupus are Pronestyl (procainamide) used to treat heart irregularities, Apresoline (hydralazine) used to treat high blood pressure, and INH (isoniazid) used to treat tuberculosis. Other drugs that can cause DILE include beta blockers, tricyclic antidepressants, penicillin, and sulfa drugs.[5]

This form of lupus is not chronic. While 90 percent of people on procainamide develop antinuclear antibodies in their blood in one year, (which signal the presence of drug-induced lupus), only 10 percent of them actually develop lupus symptoms. This form of lupus is generally quite mild and will disappear after discontinuing the prescription drug, although some people may need to be treated with lupus medications.

Discoid Lupus

This chronic form of lupus, technically called discoid lupus erythematosus (DLE) or cutaneous lupus, falls on the mild end of the lupus spectrum, affecting only the skin. A raised red rash may appear on the face, neck, ear, scalp, or elsewhere. About 10 percent of people diagnosed with lupus have this form of the disease, and only 5 to 10 percent of that group will, over time, develop systemic lupus.[6]

Neonatal Lupus

This nonchronic form of lupus is usually limited to children of mothers who carry a specific autoantibody that crosses the placenta (discussed further in chapter 7). The lupus manifestations such as rash usually disappear during the first year of life because the mothers' antibodies get

---

Let's Get Organized

Dr. Daniel J. Wallace, a former president of the Lupus Foundation of America, began working with lupus patients back in the mid-1970s, just shortly after the American College of Rheumatology first published the diagnostic criteria for this disease. He has seen the number of diagnosed patients in need of information and medical support climb, but he also recognizes few people know much about the disease. "Lupus falls short on publicity," says Dr. Wallace, "because it's considered a woman's disease, which makes it harder in certain ways to get attention and funding. The cause also lacks a major celebrity spokesperson who can give lupus much-needed attention."

Dr. Wallace is absolutely right. It is getting harder to obtain any large-scale recognition of a disease without that "endorsement." According to *Healthweek,* a PBS news program, contributions to the American Paralysis Association have more than doubled since Christopher Reeve became their spokesperson in 1995. Also in those years, federal research funding for spinal cord injuries has increased by almost $20 million—largely due to Reeve's activism and testimony on Capitol Hill.[7]

"used up" and the babies do not make more of it on their own.[8] Rarely, certain autoantibodies can cause heart damage in the electrical system of a baby's heart leading to the need for a pacemaker. (See the following section for the definitions of antibody and autoantibody.)

THE CAUSE OF LUPUS

We are all born with a built-in defense system against disease called the immune system. More than 100 million cells, each targeted toward specific viruses and bacteria, fight infection when a disease-causing virus or bacterium finds its way into the body.

Sometimes things go wrong with this system. A healthy immune system produces antibodies (special proteins that help fight and destroy invading organisms such as viruses and bacteria) to battle foreign substances. If you have lupus, however, you have an autoimmune disorder in which the immune system loses its ability to tell the difference between foreign substances and its own cells and tissues. The immune system then makes antibodies directed against the body's healthy cells and tissues. These antibodies, called autoantibodies, "attack" various parts of the body, causing inflammation, injury to tissues, and pain, producing the symptoms of lupus. (The specific autoantibodies involved in lupus are discussed in chapter 2.)

FROM SPOKESPERSON TO PATIENT

In the late 1970s, the Lupus Foundation of America asked Mary McDonough to serve as a celebrity spokesperson. You probably remember Mary best as the middle daughter, Erin, on the TV series, *The Waltons*. At the time, Mary did not have lupus, nor was there a history of the disease anywhere in her family. As a 17-year-old female, however, she represented the gender and population group likely to develop lupus, and so it was hoped she would bring attention and greater understanding to this disease. This is her story:

The Autoimmune Family

Along with lupus, a few other diseases in the autoimmune family are:

- Multiple sclerosis

- Diabetes

- Rheumatoid arthritis

- Hyperthyroidism (Graves' disease)

- The Hashimoto form of hypothyroidism

- Scleroderma

"When I became the spokesperson, I learned all I could about lupus and then began to speak about its symptoms and treatment on television and with writers for newsmagazines. How ironic, that for 10 years after I started to experience symptoms of lupus myself, at age 24, my doctors wouldn't believe that there was anything wrong with me! I think their refusal to even consider the possibility that my symptoms were signs of lupus had to do with the fact that the symptoms first began right after I had breast augmentation surgery with silicone gel implants. Within the first 24 hours, I developed a terrible rash on my chest and back. The other symptoms of chronic fatigue, achy joints, muscle pain, low-grade fever, flulike symptoms, chronic infections, headaches, dizziness, memory loss, hair loss, light sensitivity, as well as fibromyalgia, rheumatoid arthritis, and Sjögren's syndrome developed over the years. But still, there was a strong resistance in the medical community, and even by some within the lupus community to tie breast implants and lupus together.

"I'm not a scientist, but I am an expert on me, so let me say it simply: I was healthy; I got implants; I got sick. I got them out; I started to get better. This doesn't happen to all women who get breast implants and there are many women with lupus who have never had implants. But in my case, there seems to be a clear connection.

"In the ten years after I had the implants inserted, I got worse and worse. I knew something was wrong with me, even though many different doctors never diagnosed me with anything out of the ordinary. I started to feel as if I was a hypochondriac and doctors began to treat me as though I was exaggerating. This made me feel even worse. I thought, 'Maybe it is all in my head. Maybe I'm fine and I am only depressed.' So I started to go to therapy, but the symptoms still continued.

"Nothing changed until I was involved in a car accident and ruptured a disk in my back. I went to physical therapy and to a chiropractor, but because I wasn't getting better, the chiropractor said I should see an orthopedic surgeon. Ironically, after going to several doctors, it was the orthopedist who told me I had too many symptoms to attribute to a bad back. He ordered a series of laboratory tests that revealed that I had an elevated level of autoantibodies that attack the body's own cells. Finally, I had a clue that something might be wrong with me. I went to see a rheumatologist who, unfortunately, spent the next five years refusing to agree that I had lupus. She gave me shots of cortisone, but never really treated the disease.

> *I started to feel as if I was a hypochondriac and doctors began to treat me as though I was exaggerating. This made me feel even worse. I thought, "Maybe it is all in my head. Maybe I'm fine and I am only depressed."*
>
> —MARY MCDONOUGH

"While under the care of this doctor, I delivered a beautiful baby girl. But unfortunately, immediately after her birth, I went into a terrible lupus flare that no one forewarned me about or bothered to treat. I did not know at the time that the disease could flare after giving birth. I had a horrible post-birth experience lasting five months. I wasn't healing; I was exhausted; I couldn't breastfeed. I was an emotional basket case. I wasn't sleeping and I was in terrible pain. My obstetrician said I "was not adjusting well to motherhood." So, once again, I thought it was just me and I was crazy to think something was wrong. I felt like a horrible failure.

"Finally, against my doctor's advice, I had the implants removed. The surgeon found that the silicone envelopes and polyurethane foam that had covered the implants had disintegrated inside my body. All that was left was the silicone gel, surrounded by my body's own scar tissue. Finally, about a year later, when my autoantibody tests were still elevated and I had other complications, my rheumatologist finally said, 'Yes, you have lupus,' but she still had no clear plan for treating me. Obviously, it was time to move on.

"After years of suffering horrible symptoms and emotional devastation, I switched to another doctor who I believe saved my life. This is a great doctor whom I trust completely. This is so important for me and has made a big difference in my health. (For one thing, I don't feel that I'm crazy anymore!) This doctor began aggressive medication therapy and I am now much better than I've been in many years. Research on women with implants suggests that getting my implants out also helped me get better. Today, I take barely any medication at all and have maybe three or four flares a year.

"I'm lucky because I have non-organ threatening lupus and I have the ability and the energy to keep working and doing all the things I love to do. I'm acting, directing, writing, and producing so many wonderful projects. I'm working more now than I had in the past when untreated lupus made it impossible to live a normal life. But now I'm back and, in fact, when I was on an episode of the TV show *ER*, I played a person who had lupus. When the producer found out that I actually had the disease, he asked if he could advertise that fact to promote the show. People close to me told me that I should keep it a secret because they believed that once word got out, it would be the kiss of death to my career. But I just couldn't do that. One problem that all people with lupus face is the fact that the disease is not well known and it has no celebrity spokesperson. This is

> *P*eople close to me told me that I should keep my lupus a secret because they believed that once word got out, it would be the kiss of death to my career.
>
> —MARY MCDONOUGH

sad because it affects research funding and public understanding. So I'm trying to do all I can to spread the word. I'm the president of a fund-raising group called Lupus L.A. and I'm on the board of a women's health organization called the National Center for Policy Research (CPR) for Women and Families (www.center4policy.org or www.cpr4womenandfamilies.org), and I have lobbied Congress on women's health issues. Overall, I'm very thankful that I was finally correctly diagnosed and treated. That has given me back my very busy and productive life.

"It's ironic that I began my association with lupus when I was a young actress serving as a celebrity spokesperson to educate people about the disease. Who could have imagined at that time that I would be doing the same thing as an adult actress, only this time speaking from personal experience?"

THE HISTORY OF LUPUS

Although *lupus* is just recently becoming a familiar word that most people now recognize as "some sort of illness," it has been around for a very long time. Descriptive articles detailing the condition date back to Hippocrates in ancient Greece. Doctors have diagnosed lupus as we now know it—rash, arthritis, kidney inflammation—since at least the mid-nineteenth century, when modern medicine began. Here is a dateline that outlines some of the most notable events in the history of lupus:

- 1200s: Physician Rogerius coined the name *lupus* (Latin for "wolf") to describe the facial lesions resembling a wolf's bite.

- 1800: Dr. Willan, a British dermatologist, included lupus in his classification of skin diseases.

- 1851: French doctor Pierre Cazanave first used the term *lupus erythematosus*.

- Mid-1880s: Viennese physicians Ferdinand von Hebra and Moriz Kaposi suggest that lupus could be more than skin deep and affect the organs of the body as well.

- 1885–1903: Sir William Osler wrote the earliest complete treatises on lupus erythematosus that, in addition to describing such symptoms as fevers and aching, clearly showed that the central nervous, musculoskeletal, pulmonary, and cardiac systems could be part of the disease.

- 1920s–1930s: Pathologists working at Mount Sinai Hospital in New York gave the first detailed pathologic descriptions of lupus, showing how it affects kidney, heart, and lung tissues. Dr. Paul Klemperer and colleagues coined the term "collagen disease," which led to our contemporary classification of lupus as an autoimmune disorder.

- 1922: The false positive test for syphilis was recognized as a reasonably common finding in SLE.

- 1948: Mayo Clinic pathologist Malcolm Hargraves published his description of the lupus erythematosus (or LE) cell. This allowed doctors to diagnose the disease faster and more reliably. Also, Dr. Hargraves at the Mayo Clinic refined the concept of autoimmune disease and showed the LE cell to be part of the antinuclear antibody reaction. SLE could now be recognized earlier and in milder and treatable forms.

- 1949: Mayo Clinic physician Dr. Phillip Hench demonstrated that a newly discovered hormone known as cortisone could treat rheumatoid arthritis. This hormone was administered to lupus patients throughout the country and immediately showed dramatic, lifesaving results.

- 1950s: Florescent tests to detect antibodies against the nucleus of cells (antinuclear antibody [ANA] tests) are developed.

- 1960s: The prognosis for lupus sufferers improved as diagnosis improved, drugs were used more appropriately, and public awareness began to develop.

- 1980s: Clinical studies by Decker and colleagues at the National Institutes of Health demonstrated that cytotoxic drugs are effective in the treatment of lupus nephritis.[9]

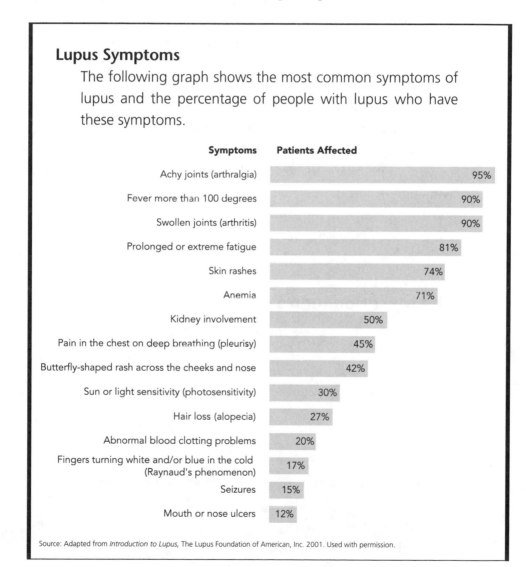

Lupus Symptoms

The following graph shows the most common symptoms of lupus and the percentage of people with lupus who have these symptoms.

Symptoms	Patients Affected
Achy joints (arthralgia)	95%
Fever more than 100 degrees	90%
Swollen joints (arthritis)	90%
Prolonged or extreme fatigue	81%
Skin rashes	74%
Anemia	71%
Kidney involvement	50%
Pain in the chest on deep breathing (pleurisy)	45%
Butterfly-shaped rash across the cheeks and nose	42%
Sun or light sensitivity (photosensitivity)	30%
Hair loss (alopecia)	27%
Abnormal blood clotting problems	20%
Fingers turning white and/or blue in the cold (Raynaud's phenomenon)	17%
Seizures	15%
Mouth or nose ulcers	12%

Source: Adapted from *Introduction to Lupus*, The Lupus Foundation of American, Inc. 2001. Used with permission.

Today, researchers continue their quest to further understand the cause, diagnosis, and treatment of lupus. See chapter 8 for the details.

THE SYMPTOMS OF LUPUS

As explained earlier, people with lupus have abnormal antibodies that cause inflammation, infection, and pain. The interesting fact about lupus that complicates this seemingly straightforward cause and effect is that the antibodies flow through the bloodstream and cause inflammation wherever they land, which can be anywhere. This is why so many different types of symptoms occur in different people. It is also difficult to state an absolute set of symptoms because most people get only a few of these symptoms and they develop almost imperceptibly over months or years. Others experience a sudden onset of symptoms, and most symptoms come and go over time. Despite this variability, there are some symptoms that are typically associated with lupus, which are explored in the following section. Although lupus can affect any part of the body, most people with lupus have symptoms in only a few organs.

The Most Common Symptoms

According to Dr. Wallace, the three most common initial symptoms of lupus are:

- Joint pain or swelling
- Skin rash
- Malaise or fatigue

Let's take a look at these early symptoms of lupus one by one.

Joint Pain or Swelling

Joint pain or swelling is a very common symptom of systemic lupus erythematosus. In fact, the Lupus Foundation of America estimates

Common Symptoms of Lupus

The most common *early* symptoms of lupus are:

- Joint pain or swelling
- Skin rash
- Malaise or fatigue

Other common symptoms of lupus are:

- Fever
- Muscle pain
- Blood disorders
- Kidney disease
- Cardiopulmonary complications
- Nervous system involvement
- Hair loss

that 95 percent of lupus cases involve achy joints.[10] Although all joints can be affected, most commonly lupus affects the fingers, wrists, elbows, shoulders, knees, and feet. The pain can occur at any time during the course of SLE, but often joint pain is present months, or even years, before the other symptoms. The degree of joint involvement varies from vague discomfort to severe lupus arthritis.

Mary Betty Stevens, M.D., of the Johns Hopkins School of Medicine in Maryland wrote a paper called "Joint and Muscle Pain in Lupus" in which she says, "Stiffness in the morning that improves as the day goes on is characteristic of lupus arthritis. Later in the day, as the individual becomes more tired, the aches may return. Another characteristic of lupus arthritis is that the pain is usually symmetrical which means that it affects similar joints on both sides of the body. Therefore, a single, chronically painful and swollen joint, even in a person who has been diagnosed with lupus, is most likely due to some other cause."[11]

The pain of lupus arthritis often comes and goes. Individual attacks may last several days or weeks and then subside, only to recur at a later date. In a small percentage of people with lupus, damage to tendons or joint coverings in the hand can occur, leading to deformity of the finger joint. But unlike rheumatoid arthritis, lupus arthritis does not cause bone or cartilage destruction.

Skin Rash

Skin rash is also very common in lupus erythematosus. The Lupus Foundation of America estimates that 74 percent of lupus cases involve skin rashes.[12] The exact cause of the skin involvement with lupus is unknown and the symptoms can range from a simple rash to itchy hives to painful and disfiguring ulcerations.

Thomas T. Provost, M.D., in the department of dermatology at the Johns Hopkins University School of Medicine, says that approximately 5 to 10 percent of patients initially presenting with only the coin-shaped lesions of discoid lupus will, with time, develop systemic features and approximately 20 percent of people with systemic lupus erythematosus will have these ring- or coin-shaped, scarring lesions as the initial symptom of their disease. The discoid lesion (characteristic of discoid lupus erythematosus) may develop thick, scaly formations or cause a thickening of the layers of underlying skin. Occasionally, discoid lupus lesions develop on the scalp, producing scarring and localized baldness (called alopecia). At times, these lesions may appear over the central portion of the face and nose, producing the characteristic butterfly rash (see figure 1.2). At the present time, research indicates that discoid lupus lesions are the result of an immunologic and inflammatory process in the skin that localizes to the skin and is not disseminated as it is in SLE.

> An estimated 95 percent of lupus cases involve achy joints, 74 percent involve skin rashes, and 81 percent involve fatigue.

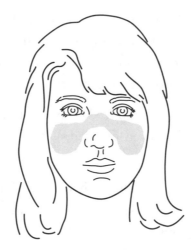

Figure 1.2—*Butterfly Rash*

A second type of skin lesion common with lupus is a non-scarring, coin-shaped red lesion, which is highly photosensitive (which means it gets worse when exposed to ultraviolet light). This type of lesion occurs in approximately 50 percent of the people who have systemic lupus erythematosus. This rash can sometimes mimic the lesions of psoriasis or it can appear as non-scarring, coin-shaped lesions. The lesions can occur on the face in a butterfly pattern or can cover large areas of the body. Unlike the discoid lupus lesions, these lesions do not produce permanent scarring or alopecia, but can still be cosmetically displeasing.[13]

According to dermatologist LindaSusan Marcus, M.D., there is no one type of skin rash that indicates lupus. "Lupus can have numerous effects on the skin," she says. "If lupus is suspected, your doctor will be looking for a number of skin abnormalities that may indicate that lupus testing is necessary, although they do not by themselves mean that lupus is present." Among numerous skin changes possible with lupus that can occur on the scalp, around the mouth, on the face, nose, mucous membranes (vagina), ears, chest, arms, or over the entire body, Dr. Marcus keeps an open eye for the following skin problems:

- Thick red papules and plaques on the head and neck (discoid lesions). There can be scarring without treatment and areas of lighter and darker pigmentation changes, as well as scale or crust, especially around the ears.

- Light-induced or sun-induced eruptions (photosensitivity) present generally on sun-exposed skin. (This is the malar or "butterfly" rash.)

- A persistent, flat or patchy, scaly red eruption (like psoriasis) with or without papules, on the upper chest, back, sides of the neck, and forearms.

- A deep inflammation with red nodules that heals with depressed scars (lupus panniculitis).

- Blistering.

- Hair loss (alopecia), which can occur in small patches or extend all over the scalp and develop in the absence of any rash.

- Hives (urticaria).

- Red, white, and blue discoloration of fingers upon exposure to cold (Raynaud's phenomenon).

Malaise or Fatigue

Malaise or fatigue is sometimes the first symptom of lupus a person notices. Malaise is that blah feeling that says something's not right. It makes you feel like canceling your plans and staying home. It makes you feel like you're coming down with the flu because you're just a little "off." But unlike most cases of occasional blahs, the malaise of lupus can be persistent and life-disruptive.

Fatigue is more severe than malaise. It is a definite and extreme sense of tiredness experienced by approximately 81 percent of people with lupus. This is not the kind of tiredness you feel after a long and active day. It is a body-draining, total depletion of stamina, for no apparent reason, that is not remedied by a good night's sleep. It is the kind of exhaustion that makes every day a struggle; it's like having a chronic case of the flu. In fact, some people say that even when their other symptoms of lupus are in remission, the fatigue remains. Naturally, you want to know, "Why do I feel so blah and tired?"

The reason for fatigue in lupus is unknown. Some people with this disease have conditions such as severe anemia, depression, hormonal problems, renal disease, or chronic fevers that can explain a degree of fatigue. But for the majority of people there is no known cause. In his article, "Lupus and Fatigue," Robert S. Schwartz, M.D., of the New England Medical Center in Massachusetts, proposes that certain brain activity may be responsible for the fatigue of lupus. He writes:

> In an autoimmune disease like systemic lupus erythematosus, the body suffers from attack by the very inflammatory mechanisms that it musters as an antimicrobial defense. One result of this is the production of small proteins of the immune system termed *lymphokines*, which signal other cells to carry out particular functions. An extremely important lymphokine is interleukin-1 (IL-1), which has many different effects on the body. Two of its important activities concern its ability to stimulate certain cells in the brain. Cells in the part of the brain called the hypothalamus respond to IL-1 by causing a rise in the body's temperature: fever. Other brain cells respond to IL-1 by producing yet another peptide that causes sleep. Injection of highly purified IL-1 will put a rabbit to sleep. Another lymphokine, TNF, has the same sleep-inducing property.
>
> Fever and rest (sleep) are part of the defense against infection. They are imposed on the patient by the body's response to the infection, which includes the production of specific fever-inducing and sleep-inducing peptide messengers. What remains to be shown is that these same mechanisms occur in the patient with active systemic lupus erythematosus—presumably they do, but actual evidence is lacking. If it is indeed true that IL-1 and TNF induce fatigue in lupus, then physicians would have at their disposal an objective means of evaluating and advising the vexed, tired lupus patient.[14]

Flares and Remissions

A **flare** is a sudden increase in symptoms. This exacerbation can be activated by common triggers such as sunlight, certain chemicals or medications, or a simple cold or flu.

A **remission** is a disease-free period. This can happen without apparent cause or be induced by medications, and can last for as short as a few days to as long as a lifetime.

Both flares and remissions are very common in lupus.

Other Common Symptoms

There are other symptoms and conditions also often experienced by people with lupus. Some of the more common include: fever, muscle pain, blood disorders, kidney disease, cardiopulmonary complications, nervous system involvement, and hair loss.

Fever

Many people with lupus have a chronic low-grade fever one to two degrees above normal. Without any other obvious infectious cause, this is generally a sign of the infectious or inflammatory process typically found in lupus.

Muscle Pain

Most people with lupus feel some muscle pain or weakness. Trunk muscles (neck, pelvic girdle and thighs, shoulder and upper arms) are the first to be affected. They might first burn, then become painful and then weak.

Inflammation of the muscles (called myositis) is found in approximately 15 percent of people with lupus.[15] Unlike the joints, the muscles can be seriously damaged by SLE, causing muscle weakness and loss of strength, unless early and appropriate treatment is given.

Blood Disorders

Dr. Schwartz says that it is not unusual for the initial signs of lupus to appear in the blood. "In some patients with lupus, a blood disorder is the primary symptom of the disease. The major hematological symptoms of SLE are anemia, thrombocytopenia (low platelet count), clotting disturbances, and low white blood cell counts."[16] Dr. Schwartz explains these blood disorders as follows:

Anemia is a reduction in the number of red blood cells. The severity of the anemia is usually proportional to the severity of a person's lupus. The fatigue suffered by many people with active lupus can often be attributed in part to anemia.

Thrombocytopenia is a low platelet count. Platelets are tiny particles in the blood that are essential for blood clotting. A severe deficiency often leads to excessive bruising of the skin or bleeding from the gums, nose, intestines, or other

> *In some patients with lupus, a blood disorder is the primary symptom of the disease.*
>
> —ROBERT S. SCHWARTZ, M.D.

organs. Pinpoint hemorrhages in the skin, called purpura, are a typical sign of thrombocytopenia. The most common cause of thrombocytopenia in people with lupus is immune thrombocytopenia. Often referred to as ITP, this is caused by antibodies against platelets. Indeed, ITP may be the dominant or even sole symptom of lupus in some patients. In rare cases, ITP and autoimmune hemolytic anemia occur together. The antibodies destroy the platelets in a manner similar to the destruction of red blood cells in autoimmune hemolytic anemia.

Clotting disturbances occur in some people with SLE when they produce an antiphospholipid antibody, specifically the lupus anticoagulant antibody. Studies suggest that the presence of this antibody increases the risk of stroke and heart attack. The term *anticoagulant* usually refers to an agent that interferes with normal blood clotting mechanisms and results in abnormal or heavy bleeding. But, the lupus anticoagulant is almost never associated with abnormal bleeding, even after injury or surgery. On the contrary, some patients with lupus anticoagulant tend to form clots abnormally, especially in veins, which results in a condition called venous thrombosis. There is currently no explanation for this paradox. The condition is generally treated with anticoagulant drugs. The presence of other antibodies to phospholipids can be associated with pregnancy loss and neurologic disorders.

Low white blood cell counts may be a sign of lupus. Generally, these abnormalities are harmless and do not cause symptoms. Occasionally, however, severely low counts of white blood cells called granulocytes can occur and result in susceptibility to bacterial infections. These cases are usually caused by lupus itself or a reaction to medication. If it is due to lupus, treatment of the inflammation leads to normalization of the white count. Treatment with antibiotics is necessary if there is infection. If a drug is the culprit, it should be discontinued.

Kidney Disease

Approximately 50 percent of people with lupus will have some degree of kidney involvement. About one-third will develop a kidney disease called lupus nephritis (*nephritis* means "inflammation of the kidney").[17]

There are few signs or symptoms of lupus nephritis. In his article "Kidney Disease and Lupus," John H. Klippel, M.D., of the Musculoskeletal and Skin Diseases, National Institutes of Health, notes that lupus nephritis does not produce pain in the abdomen or back, and it doesn't cause pain or burning during urination. But the loss of protein in the urine from lupus nephritis can lead to fluid retention with weight gain and swelling (edema), which can result in puffiness in the legs, ankles, or fingers. This puffiness is often the first symptom of lupus nephritis. Other signs include pink urine, high blood pressure, headache, or bloody nose.[18]

The course of kidney disease varies from person to person. In some, the urine abnormalities are very mild and may be present in one urine study and absent from the next. This form is rather common and generally does not require any special medical evaluation or treatment. In some patients, however, the abnormal findings on urine studies persist or may even worsen over time. People with this type of lupus nephritis are at risk for loss of kidney function. If not treated properly, toxins or poisons that would normally be filtered out of the blood by the kidneys can build up in the body, causing a deteriorating physical condition and eventual death.

Although kidney disease is a common component of lupus, Dr. Klippel cautions that not all kidney problems in people with lupus are due to lupus nephritis. "For instance," he says, "infections of the urinary tract with burning on urina-

> *Approximately 50 percent of people with lupus will have some degree of kidney involvement.*

tion are quite common in lupus patients and require antibiotic treatment. Similarly, medications used in lupus treatment can produce signs or symptoms of kidney disease that can be confused with lupus nephritis. Salicylate compounds (for example, aspirin), or non-steroidal anti-inflammatory drugs are the most common type of medications used by lupus patients that can produce kidney problems. These drugs can cause loss of kidney function or fluid retention. These problems usually fade when the medications are discontinued."[19]

Tiffany, 25, who works for an advertising agency, has had kidney nephritis directly related to her lupus, but fortunately she is under the care of a very knowledgeable physician and the tissue inflammation is now under control. "A few months after I was diagnosed with lupus, my doctor did a urinalysis and it showed an abundance of red blood cells, and so then I had a kidney biopsy that showed severe kidney inflammation. My kidneys were functioning, but they would have shut down pretty soon if my doctor didn't act quickly. Detecting kidney disease early is key to living a normal life, so I'm very grateful that it was diagnosed right away."

Cardiopulmonary Complications

The heart and lungs are frequently affected by lupus. The degree varies from having no symptoms at all to having life-threatening complications. Since the degree of inflammation is difficult to judge by symptoms alone, you should not ignore any chest pain or discomfort.

Normally functioning lungs effortlessly exchange oxygen for carbon dioxide. If you have lupus, you may experience a variety of lung problems that can interfere with this process, including shortness of breath, chest pain, rapid breathing, fever, or cough. The most common lung complications associated with lupus are pleurisy and pneumonitis.

Pleurisy is the chest pain that occurs when the lining of the lung (the pleura) becomes inflamed. Elliot Chartash, M.D., of Cornell University Medical College, explains that the pleura is a membrane that covers the outside of the lung and the inside of the chest cavity. It produces a small amount of fluid to lubricate the space between the lung and the chest wall. If you have lupus, the autoantibodies may attack this membrane, causing it to become inflamed (a condition called pleuritis). This is the most common lung complication associated with lupus.[20]

Dr. Chartash says that the symptoms of pleuritis include severe, often sharp, stabbing pain, which may be located in a specific area or areas of the chest. The pain is often made worse by taking a deep breath, coughing, sneezing, or laughing. Analgesics, nonsteroidal anti-inflammatory drugs (NSAIDs), or corticosteroids can be used to treat this condition.[21]

Pneumonitis is inflammation within the lung tissue, which can be caused by an infection or by lupus. Dr. Chartash writes:

Infection is the most common cause of pneumonitis in people with lupus. Bacteria, viruses, fungi, or protozoa are organisms that can cause infection in the lung. Sometimes pneumonitis may occur without infection and is then called noninfectious or lupus pneumonitis. Since both forms of pneumonitis have the same symptoms—fever, chest pain, shortness of breath, and cough—the patient is assumed to have an infection until proven otherwise. Treatment of pneumonitis initially includes a course of antibiotics. If laboratory and other diagnostic tests show no proof of infection, then the diagnosis is likely lupus pneumonitis. This noninfectious pneumonitis is treated with high doses of corticosteroids. Immunosuppressive drugs may be added if the inflammation is not controlled with steroids.[22]

Chest pain associated with lupus also can be caused by inflammation of several components of the heart. If the pericardium (the sac surrounding the heart) is attacked by autoantibodies and becomes inflamed, the resulting pericarditis causes sharp chest pain underneath the sternum with breathing, fever, rapid heartbeat, and occasionally shortness of breath. It is estimated that about 25 percent of people with lupus experience this complication.[23] This, like pleuritis, usually responds to NSAIDs or low to moderate doses of steroids.

If the muscle layer of the heart (the myocardium) becomes inflamed, the symptoms can include rapid heartbeat, an abnormal electrocardiogram, an irregular heartbeat, and, rarely, heart failure. Significant heart muscle disease is not common in lupus, however.

If the lining of the inside of the heart (the endocardium) becomes inflamed, the heart valves can be damaged, but this rarely affects the pumping efficiency of the heart. Rarely does the inflammation and scarring of valves lead to a deformity requiring valve replacement. If you have systemic lupus and chest pain, your physician will be alert for valvular heart disease.

Finally, lupus can cause the coronary arteries to become prematurely narrowed, interfering with the body's ability to deliver blood and oxygen to the heart muscle. Cholesterol deposits inside the artery wall (atherosclerosis) are the most common cause of coronary artery disease in lupus. Research suggests that lupus patients receiving steroids have a higher risk of developing atherosclerosis, but its evolution is also hastened by high cholesterol levels, SLE inflammation itself, and possibly antiphospholipid antibodies. Thus, optimal control of all of these factors is mandatory.[24]

Nervous System Involvement

Nervous system involvement in people with systemic lupus erythematosus may manifest as headaches, confusion, difficulty with concentration, fatigue, and occasionally seizures, strokes, or other signs. The potential causes include lupus itself, blood clots due to antiphospholipid antibodies, and other medical problems such as infections, severe hypertension, or abnormalities in blood chemistry. It is thought that, as with any other tissue, the tissues of the nervous system can become a target for lupus autoantibodies. When antibodies attack the brain, cerebritis (inflammation of the brain) may result. Although temporary, this can cause significant disability. If scarring occurs, the damage can be permanent and leave a patient with lasting effects.[25]

> *Nervous system involvement in people with SLE may manifest as headaches, confusion, difficulty with concentration, fatigue, and occasionally seizures or strokes.*

Dr. Wallace wrote a paper called "Systemic Lupus and the Nervous System" in which he discusses how lupus can affect the nervous system. The following information is from this article.[26]

The central nervous system (CNS, which consists of the brain and spinal cord) and the peripheral nervous system (which is comprised of nerve fibers that supply the skin and muscles with the power needed for sensation and movement) are most often involved in SLE.

Symptoms of central nervous system disease due to lupus itself include CNS vasculitis, cognitive dysfunction, and lupus headache.

CNS vasculitis is inflammation of the blood vessels of the brain. It occurs in up to 10 percent of all lupus patients and is the only form of CNS disease that is included in the American College of Rheumatology criteria for defining SLE. Characterized by high fevers, headache, lethargy or abnormal mental function, stroke or seizures, and meningitis-like stiffness of the neck, it can rapidly progress to stupor and coma if not aggressively managed. CNS vasculitis is the most serious effect of SLE and usually requires hospitalization and rapid control of inflammation with high doses of corticosteroids and possibly immunosuppressive drugs.

Cognitive dysfunction affects up to 50 percent of people with lupus at some point in the course of the illness. These people describe feelings of confusion, memory impairment, and difficulty expressing their thoughts. This collection of symptoms is most often found in people with mild to moderately active SLE. Spinal taps, brain wave tests (EEGs), magnetic resonance imaging (MRI), or computerized tomography (CT) scans of the brain may all be normal, but these symptoms can be clearly documented by neuropsychological testing and a neurodiagnostic test called the positron emission tomography (PET) scan which shows blood flow abnormalities. The reason for these symptoms is not known, but it may have something to do with changes in how a group of chemicals known as cytokines are handled or it may be related to certain parts of the brain not getting enough oxygen.

> Cognitive dysfunction—feelings of confusion, memory impairment, and difficulty expressing one's thoughts—affects up to 50 percent of people with lupus at some point in the course of the illness.

Twenty-six-year-old salesclerk, Jennie, often finds cognitive dysfunction the most difficult part of her day. "Last week," she says, "I was trying to give a 10 percent discount on $37.50 and I kept thinking the total cost would be $7.50. Even though I knew that couldn't be right, I just couldn't figure out what was wrong. I had to finally ask for help. I came home in tears not really because of the mistake, but because I'm not sure what is happening to me. I concentrate really hard and I still make mistakes and I come home totally exhausted. Some days it's just so hard."

Lupus headaches (similar to migraine pain) affect approximately 20 percent of people with SLE. PET scans indicate abnormalities in blood vessel tone or the ability of a vessel to dilate or constrict. Lupus headache is treated like tension headaches or migraine, although corticosteroids are occasionally useful.

Symptoms of peripheral nervous system lupus are varied and depend on which nerves are involved. Involvement of the cranial nerves in the head can cause visual disturbances, facial pain, drooping of the eyelid(s), ringing in the ear(s), and dizziness. Inflammation of the blood vessels supplying the peripheral nerves can lead to symptoms of numbness, tingling, or weakness in the arms or legs. Occasionally, loss of sensation or muscular weakness in the fingers can occur due to a pinched nerve in the wrist (as happens in carpal tunnel syndrome).

Of course, peripheral nervous system symptoms may be due to conditions other than lupus. Electrical studies, such as electromyo-gram (EMG) and nerve conduction tests are usually helpful in deter-mining if symptoms are due to some other cause such as a herniated disc or a metabolic abnormality as in diabetes. Inflammation of pe-ripheral nerves is treated with corticosteroids.

Hair Loss

About 30 percent of people with systemic or discoid lupus experience significant hair loss (alopecia).[27] Some experience diffuse fallout, while others lose hair in patches around the scalp. Some notice a gen-eralized thinning of the hair. Although the exact reason for these symptoms is unclear, there are three strong possibilities:

- Inflammatory cells may attack the hair follicles under the scalp.
- Medications such as chemotherapeutic agents and steroids have been known to cause hair loss.
- Miscellaneous causes such as infection, chemotherapy, emo-tional stress, and hormonal imbalances may also play a role.

Hair loss all over the body (alopecia totalis) has been known to occur in lupus. Fortunately, in most cases, all hair begins to grow again spontaneously.

LUPUS TRIGGERS

So now you know that lupus is caused by an autoimmune response that can attack many cells, tissues, organs, and systems of the body, producing a wide range of symptoms. But still, questions remain:

What causes the body's immune system to go haywire and attack itself? Why do some people struggle with lupus all their lives, and others have never even heard of it? Why does the disease seem to go into remission and then flare without warning? These are all good questions—without any clear answers. There are many possibilities but no absolutes, because what triggers the disease in one person may have absolutely no effect on another. What causes one person with lupus to have a major flare may leave another person untouched. You will have to pay close attention to the patterns of your unique disease to try to uncover what triggers affect you and under what circum-

> *You will have to pay close attention to the patterns of your unique disease to try to uncover what triggers affect you and under what circumstances.*

stances. A few suspected triggers known to induce, aggravate, or accelerate lupus include infections, chemical factors, ultraviolet light, certain medications, stress, and perhaps genetics.

Chemical Factors

There are certain chemical factors that are known to occasionally play a role in initiating lupus or making it worse. In *The Lupus Book*, Dr. Wallace writes:

> Aromatic amines are the chemical agents that may induce or aggravate rheumatic disease. This class includes hair-coloring solutions, hydrazines (e.g., tobacco smoke), and tartrazines (e.g., food colorings or medication preservatives). Aromatic amines are broken down in the body by a process known as acetylation. An increased incidence of drug-induced lupus has been observed after exposure to aromatic amines in patients who are slow acetylators, or those who metabolize aromatic amines slowly. About half of all Americans are slow acetylators. The mechanism by which aromatic amines may induce an immunologic reaction is poorly understood, and only a small percentage of people exposed to these chemicals ever develop clinical immune disease.[28]

As we saw in the case of Mary McDonough, chemicals such as silicone gel implanted into the body may trigger lupus. Although there are no studies yet to support the relationship between breast implants and lupus, still, the possibility exists that many chemical toxins (not yet fully identified) can influence the course of lupus. The best thing you can do is to keep alert to the possible association between your contact with a chemical substance and the onset or flare of lupus.

Ultraviolet Light

Some people who have lupus are very sensitive to the sun's rays. That is why the overwhelming majority of lupus skin lesions occur on sun-exposed areas. In addition, because ultraviolet radiation is thought to increase the response of the immune system, exposure to too much ultraviolet light can precipitate or aggravate a flare-up for many people with lupus. And what's more, about 90 percent of people with systemic or discoid lupus who have the suspect antibodies are photosensitive, meaning they burn very easily.[29]

There are many studies that find an especially strong relationship between sun exposure and the skin lesions of lupus. One study has shown that ultraviolet light in both the sunburn light spectrum and the long-wavelength light spectrum (those wavelengths that are not blocked by window glass) will cause lupus lesions to appear on the skin of people with systemic lupus erythematosus, those with the lesions of subacute cutaneous lupus, and also on those who have only scarring lupus lesions (discoid lesions) with no evidence of systemic disease.[30]

Obviously, given this information, you should be cautious about direct sun exposure. As with many lupus triggers, however, not everyone will react the same. Some people with lupus report having no reaction at all to sunlight and others find that even the slightest amount of sunlight can cause them great fatigue, pain, and skin rash. To help yourself manage your symptoms, you might keep a journal to track how you feel when you spend a day in the sun compared to when you stay out of the sun completely.

Lupus Triggers

The most common factors that can trigger the onset or the exacerbation of lupus include:

- Chemicals found in certain hair-coloring solutions, tobacco smoke, food colorings, and medication preservatives
- Ultraviolet light (sunlight)
- Medications, including some sulfa-based drugs, antibiotics, and synthetic hormones
- Stress
- Bacteria and viruses
- Genetics

Medications

As discussed earlier in this chapter, over 70 prescription medications are known to bring on drug-induced lupus erythematosus. When the drugs are withdrawn, the disease disappears. Those who have systemic lupus erythematosus, however, often find that certain drugs can cause a preexisting lupus to flare up. Most of the trigger drugs cause the flare by acting as sun-sensitizing agents or by promoting hypersensitivity or allergy-like reactions. The drugs that most commonly trigger lupus flares are sulfa-based drugs, antibiotics, and synthetic hormones.

Sulfa-based drugs and antibiotics. Some antidiabetic drugs (sulfonylureas), rheumatoid arthritis drugs (sulfasalazine), and diuretics (thiazides and furosemide) contain sulfa and can cause a lupus flare. Sulfonamide-based antibiotics Bactrim or Septra (commonly prescribed to women with urinary tract infections) as well as the antibiotics penicillin and some tetracyclines are also known to cause photosensitivity and can cause a flare in some people.[31]

Hormones. Oral contraceptives and hormone replacement therapies containing high doses of estrogen can exacerbate SLE. This complication rarely occurs with today's low-dose estrogen- or progesterone-containing compounds, however.

Since there is such a strong link between these drugs and lupus, you should always ask your physician or pharmacist to help you avoid medications high in sulfa or estrogen and those that cause photosensitivity.

Stress

Stress, emotional upset, physical trauma, and fatigue cannot cause lupus. But for those who are predisposed to lupus, these factors can trigger onset and flare. The negative effects of stress on the body are well known. It affects blood pressure, heart rate, respiration, metabolism, circulation, and muscle tension, and there is little doubt that all this can alter the optimal functioning of the immune system. That is probably why doctors who treat lupus have seen patients whose disease has spread to other organs or who had severe inflammatory joint reactions after serious emotional trauma, surgery, or motor vehicle accidents.

Doctors have seen lupus patients whose disease has spread to other organs or who had severe inflammatory joint reactions after serious emotional trauma, surgery, or motor vehicle accidents.

Tiffany (whom you met earlier when she talked about her kidney disease) was diagnosed with systemic lupus erythematosus one year ago, shortly after the sudden death of her father. "My doctor told me that stress is definitely linked to lupus," she recalls. "High levels for a long time, or stress that isn't channeled properly can spark autoimmune diseases and can flare up lupus. This was a very stressful time for me. My father was a healthy man who died without warning from a heart attack in January. He lived in New York State and I was up in Boston when he died. I didn't know about his death (I just thought he was sick) until I arrived at the hospital and my mother told me. I couldn't believe it. The funeral was in early February, but we couldn't bury him until May when the snow was gone and the ground thawed. This really dragged things out and I couldn't find closure for so long. Between his death and his burial, I was back at work trying to keep up in this very hectic and fast-paced career in advertising. That just added to the stress, and then I got engaged (which is a good thing, but still stressful!).

"That June I felt the first symptoms of lupus when I got swollen fingers and painful wrist joints. I went to the doctor in July and he was very quick to take blood tests for lupus and Lyme disease and he told me right away that I had lupus. I'm not sure if stress was the sole trigger for my lupus, but it seems obvious to me that the two are connected. So much was going on in my life at that time."

Genetics

Our environment is full of possible lupus triggers, but only a small percentage of the people with lupus respond negatively to each one. This fact suggests that lupus results when a specific predisposing set of genes is exposed to the right combination of factors that influence the risk of getting and exacerbating lupus.

Researchers now believe that there are various inherited genes that predispose a person to respond to certain triggers and develop lupus. In about 5 percent of the people with lupus, a single gene may be responsible, but for the other 95 percent, multiple genes are required. Some authorities estimate that a minimum of three or four, and possibly as many as six, susceptibility genes are required.[32]

Even though researchers have not yet isolated these "lupus genes," there is no doubt that certain genetic markers are linked with the specific autoantibodies associated with lupus. For example, although lupus is not contagious and no known specific bacterium or virus causes it, it appears that those genetically predisposed to lupus can have the process turned on by various viruses or bacteria. The evidence for this stems from the finding of elevated levels of viral antibodies in certain patients, virus particles in lupus tissue, and documentation that microbes can mimic foreign substances or antigens that turn on autoimmunity.[33] This is why after a bout of the flu or even the common cold, you may have your initial lupus symptoms or experience a lupus flare, while others suffering the same flu or cold will have no lupus response ever.

If you have lupus, members of your immediate family (brothers, sisters, parents, and children) are at a slightly increased risk for developing it, too. Several surveys have estimated this risk at 10 percent for your daughter and 2 percent for your son.[34] Your brother or sister has a twentyfold increased risk of developing SLE compared with the general population.[35]

But there are many cases of lupus in which there is no known inherited, genetic link. Many experts feel that in these cases, however, it is likely that there are other diseases in the family that are related to lupus. These are usually autoimmune diseases such as Sjögren's syndrome, rheumatoid arthritis, low platelet disorders, or various kinds of anemia.[36]

> *If you have lupus, members of your immediate family (brothers, sisters, parents, and children) are at a slightly increased risk for developing it, too.*

Although your physician can't explain exactly why your immune system attacks your own body, you can help yourself avoid a flare by keeping track of these known triggers and monitoring what you've been doing, what you've eaten, what medicines you've taken, and where you've been just before your symptoms flared. This is one area of your disease management in which you have a strong role to play.

WHO GETS LUPUS?

You're probably tired of people asking you, "What's lupus?" It's true that lupus is not well known or understood by many people, but according to the Lupus Foundation of America, more people have lupus

---

Lipstick and Lupus?

The possible triggers of lupus are many, but probably not as many as some Web sites, books, alternative healers, and other people with the disease might tell you. Even medically sound research has hit quite a few dead ends. A widely cited report, published 25 years ago, speculating that lipstick could trigger lupus attacks has caused much concern and speculation. But follow-up studies have shown that there is no such connection.[37] Today, there is worry about microwaves, aspartame artificial sweetener, and various other triggers, all without any evidence. Look for reproducible scientific validity before you accept as fact the things you read or hear.

---

than AIDS, cerebral palsy, multiple sclerosis, sickle-cell anemia, and cystic fibrosis *combined*. LFA market research data indicates that between 1.4 and 2 million people have reported being diagnosed with lupus.[38] Obviously, you are not alone and this is not a rare disease.

Lupus by Race

In the United States, lupus has been found to be more prevalent in African Americans, Latinos, Native Americans, and Asians. There are certain countries where the disease is quite common, such as China, Cambodia, and Thailand.[39]

Although some medical experts feel that the research on Native Americans and Asians is still in need of further scientific corroboration, studies such as the one by the Oklahoma Medical Research Foundation have found that SLE occurs four times more often in female African Americans than in white women.[40] For this reason, many medical professionals feel there is a need to bring more awareness and support services into African American communities.

Lupus in Women

Although lupus may affect people of either sex, females are at greatest risk for developing the systemic form of the disease. In those diagnosed between the ages of 15 and 45, close to 90 percent are women, which explains why lupus is sometimes called "a woman's disease." The fact that lupus cases are far more common during the childbearing years and less common before puberty and after menopause, and that symptoms are often worse immediately before menstruation and during or after pregnancy, have led many to believe that female sex hormones, particularly estrogen, influence the immune system, making females more susceptible.[41]

Lupus in Men

Only about 10 percent of the people with lupus are men. This may make this group feel "odd" or even "less masculine," but there is no evidence at all that lupus is the result of a diminished degree of "manliness." Men with lupus are perfectly normal males. They have normal voices, hair patterns, muscles, sexual drive and performance, fertility, and other typically "male" characteristics. Homosexuality is

Statistical Facts

Here are a few statistics you might find interesting:

- Although lupus can first appear at any age, the most common time for the onset is between the ages of 15 and 45.

- Roughly 50,000 new cases are diagnosed each year.

- Lupus strikes no less than one person out of every 2,000 in the total population.[42]

no more common among people with lupus than it is among the population as a whole.[43] More men than women develop drug-induced lupus because the medications that produce drug-induced lupus are used more frequently in men than in women.[44] The symptoms, treatment, progression, and prognosis for lupus are the same in both males and females.

Lupus in the Elderly

There are two groups of elderly people with lupus: those who have been diagnosed with the disease years earlier and those who are diagnosed after the age of 55. Although drug-induced lupus is not uncommon in patients over age 55 (because the causative drugs are commonly prescribed to this group), very few develop systemic lupus erythematosus after age 55. Those who do are as likely to be male as female.

Some studies have found that SLE in those over age 50 is generally milder, with more pleurisy, pericarditis, and arthritis and less kidney and central nervous system complications than usually occur in lupus in the general population. Not all studies agree, however. Some find a poorer prognosis for the elderly, but many feel this may be because the disease is not diagnosed in the elderly early enough to provide the proper treatment needed for a good outcome.[45] Also, older people have other medical problems that can have an impact on the outcome.

> *More men than women develop drug-induced lupus because the medications that produce drug-induced lupus are used more frequently in men than in women.*

Lupus in Children

Neonatal lupus, which affects newborns, is different from SLE that affects children. Neonatal lupus can cause heart defects or temporary skin lesions in some babies born to mothers with SLE. As stated previously, this illness is due to the presence of certain antibodies passed

Famous People with Lupus

- Flannery O'Connor, the novelist credited with creating the Southern Gothic genre, died in 1964 of kidney failure caused by lupus.

- Charles Kuralt, one of the most well-loved journalists of the twentieth century, died in 1997 of complications from lupus.

- Jill Furtado, a member of the U.S. Olympic ski team and mountain bike world champion, was diagnosed with lupus in 1997, after being initially misdiagnosed with Lyme disease.

- Grammy award–winning entertainer Seal (best known for his songs "Kiss from a Rose" and "Fly Like an Eagle") was diagnosed with lupus in 1986 and bears facial scars from the disease.

from the mother to child, rather than from biological disturbances within the child. The symptoms will degrade and disappear gradually during the first year of life.[46]

However, true systemic lupus erythematosus may develop in children between the age of 3 and the onset of puberty. This form of lupus is usually a severe, organ-threatening disease, but fortunately accounts for less than 5 percent of all lupus cases.[47] In an article entitled "Lupus and Kids," Malcolm P. Rogers, M.D., associate professor of psychiatry at Harvard Medical School in Massachusetts, states that childhood lupus is essentially the same disease as found in adults. "Joint pain appears to be the most common complaint," he says, "and fever, fatigue, and a butterfly rash are also common. As with adults, kidney involvement is one of the more serious manifestations of lupus."[48]

Like any child with a chronic illness, children with lupus are at risk for emotional and social problems. Jimmy Lawrence, M.D., chief of rheumatology at the Nemours Children's Clinic in Pensacola, Florida, treats many children with lupus and other chronic conditions and he says, "Even when the condition is stabilized, these children are condemned to daily medications, ongoing doctor visits and medical testing. They are aware that they are different from their siblings and friends; they are often in pain and they experience negative side effects from their medications, and they know their parents are worried." In an ideal world, Dr. Lawrence feels that every one of these kids would have professional counseling to help them learn to live with a chronic condition. "But," he says, "the next best thing is to find a support group. If your child had asthma, he or she would know other children dealing with the same problem. But it's unlikely that your child (or you!) knows anyone else with this illness. You both need to talk to other kids and families who are taking the same medications, who are finding ways to live with lupus, and who understand your worries."

In the end, all is not bad news. "Parents have to understand that this is not a death sentence," cautions Dr. Lawrence. "It's hard work to get through the ups and downs of chronic illness, but based on medical evidence, I'm very optimistic about the future for kids with lupus."

THE EXPECTED COURSE OF LUPUS

Mild (non-organ threatening) lupus occasionally disappears spontaneously. But in almost all cases, systemic lupus erythematosus is a chronic, incurable disease. Although there have been some rare cases of spontaneous remission (especially rare in organ-threatening disease), Dr. Wallace tells us that complete disappearance of lupus in the heart, lung, kidney, liver, or blood systems is so rare that when it happens it can be called a miracle. In fact, he says, "When one well-documented patient with severe lupus prayed to Father Junipero Serra (founder of the Spanish missions in California in the 1700s) and had her organ-threatening disease disappear, this evidence was submitted to the Vatican, where Father Serra was (and still is) being considered for sainthood."[49]

Still, the prognosis for those with lupus is positive. Your chances of living a full, normal life have improved significantly over the last several decades. Dr. Wallace informs us that the first lupus survival study done in 1939 found that half of the patients in the study were dead within 2 years of diagnosis; in 1955, half of the patients were dead within 4 years; and in 1969, within 10 years. Today, more than 90 percent of all lupus patients live more than 10 years.[50] In fact, the Lupus Foundation of America tells us that 80 to 90 percent of the people with lupus can look forward to a normal life span.[51]

These encouraging statistics rely heavily on personal involvement. You will need to find the right doctor and form a close partnership, understand your treatments, and work hard to keep yourself healthy. The following chapters will show you how to do this.

CHAPTER 2

Diagnosis

❧

THERE'S GOOD NEWS on the diagnosis front: Unlike 20 years ago, you can now probably get the correct diagnosis of lupus without spending years going for test after test after test and being told in the end that you just need to learn to relax. Today, lupus is recognized as an autoimmune disease with specific diagnostic criteria and treatment protocols.

The bad news is that not all doctors are familiar with these protocols and, even in the most experienced hands, the diagnosis is still a tricky one that in some cases takes time, effort, and patience to establish. If a person goes to her general practitioner with achy joints, she may be treated for arthritis. Then a year later, her dentist may suggest a medicated rinse for the mouth sores she's developed, and a few months later, she may end up at the dermatologist for a skin rash. Each doctor is appropriately treating her symptoms, but she needs one of them to look at the total health picture to put the pieces together and think to test her for lupus.

If you suspect that you may have lupus and are reading this chapter to find out how you can be sure, it's important for you to know that you can play a leading role in this process. You need to keep track of your symptoms and your test results over time. You need to tell

Self-Test for Lupus

Before you begin the time-consuming search for the right doctor and the right diagnosis, you might want to answer the following questions:

1. Have you ever had arthritis or rheumatism for more than 3 months?

2. Do your fingers become pale, numb, or uncomfortable in the cold?

3. Have you had any sores in your mouth for more than 2 weeks?

4. Have you been told that you have low blood counts (anemia, low white cell count, or low platelet count)?

5. Have you ever had a prominent rash on your checks for more than a month?

6. Does your skin break out after you have been in the sun (not sunburn)?

7. Has it ever been painful for more than a few days to take a deep breath (pleurisy)?

8. Have you ever been told you have protein in your urine?

9. Have you ever had a seizure, convulsion, or fit?

If you answer "yes" to at least three of these questions, there's a possibility you have lupus and should be tested for the disease.

Source: "Test Yourself for Lupus," Lupus Foundation of American, Inc., 2001. Used with permission.

your doctor your full medical history. Don't downplay symptoms that come and go (such as swollen fingers or fatigue). You are your own best advocate, so take charge, gather information from this chapter and from other readings, and give your doctor all the information needed to make an accurate diagnosis.

As there are still some doctors who are not familiar with the symptoms of lupus or who may not be sure how to diagnose this disease, you should bring this information with you to your general practitioner to back up your concern and point your medical care in the right direction.

THE REASON FOR ALL THE CONFUSION

Lupus is not easy to diagnose, even for rheumatologists who specialize in this area of medicine. There are three primary reasons for the difficulty: There is no one test that can positively say for sure if you have lupus or not; in the early stages of the disease, lupus can be difficult to distinguish from other connective tissue disorders such as rheumatoid arthritis; and positive blood and laboratory test results may or may not mean lupus, or may or may not mean other diseases instead or as well.

This third point about positive test results is especially perplexing. If your antinuclear (ANA) test (a common test for suspected lupus explained later in this chapter) is positive, for example, this is a strong indication that you may have lupus. But a positive ANA result is also found in patients with other conditions such as rheumatoid arthritis. To muddy the water even more, just because you have rheumatoid arthritis doesn't mean you don't also have lupus and vice versa. So diagnosing your painful joints as arthritis shouldn't automatically rule out the possibility of lupus.

Both you and your doctor will need to be patient and persistent to correctly analyze all your symptoms and test results. Remember, the diagnosis of lupus is based upon your clinical presentation of symptoms (such as joint pain and fatigue) and upon signs (warm and swollen joints, low platelet count), not solely on the basis of the ANA test. The test is always placed in the context of your medical presentation.

A TALE OF MISDIAGNOSIS

During the diagnosis process, many people have struggled to remain hopeful. Eugene is one of them. "I had the symptoms of lupus for years and years," Eugene remembers, "but my doctor couldn't figure out what was wrong because my blood tests didn't show anything. So I took about four aspirins every day for the aches and pains without knowing exactly what I had and that seemed to help me get by. Then things changed back in 1993 when I was 57 years old. I had problems with my prostate and went to my family physician. When my blood work came back, the doctor called me and said that my liver function was way off. He thought maybe the test results were wrong, so he repeated the tests and they came up even worse the second time. He didn't know what was going on, but after more and more tests, he felt I should have my gallbladder taken out. So I did, but of course that didn't improve the liver function. I also went to a gastrointestinal specialist in my area who did an endoscopy to check out the digestive system, looking for blocks that could be interfering with the liver functioning, but he, too, found nothing wrong.

"By this time, I had swollen glands in my neck, shoulder area, and groin, and I was losing a lot of weight, so I decided to go to a well-known medical center about 45 miles south of my home and try new doctors. A gastroenterologist there gave me a physical exam, ordered lots of blood work and a whole battery of tests, and told me that I had an enlarged liver and spleen. He and all his four associates agreed that I had a form of cancer called lymphoma. They sent me to an oncologist.

"At this point, I had lost 33 pounds and my health was really failing. This doctor did a biopsy of my lymph glands and the results came back negative. Then I went for another biopsy of different glands. Again, the results were negative. After the second time, the surgeon said I didn't have cancer, but the oncologist insisted that I did, but he just hadn't found exactly where it was yet. He did notice, however, that my blood platelet count was extremely low, so he put me on the drug prednisone. Within five months, my glands shrunk, my blood platelet count went way up, and I was feeling much better. The oncologist said the prednisone was effective against some cancers and this was the result. (He just wouldn't give up the cancer idea.) After I weaned off the medication, the symptoms began to return.

"While the doctors were still arguing among themselves, my family was sure that I wasn't going to live to the end of the year. I was still going for tests twice a week and giving eight or nine blood samples. Then I had two CAT scans done that showed a swelling in my stomach. At that time, the oncologist wanted to do surgery to examine the swollen tissue (where he was sure he'd find the cancer) and remove my spleen. But my wife and I had had enough and I wasn't going to have this surgery based on vague suspicions."

Despite all these dead ends and "vague suspicions," Eugene didn't give up. He continued his search for a diagnosis. "I then went to an infectious disease doctor and had another whole battery of tests. He even tested me for AIDS. (I'm just glad he didn't test for syphilis; that would have been devastating to get the false positive that lupus can cause, especially since no one knew what they were doing to begin with.) At the end of all the testing, this doctor wasn't confident that the swollen lymph glands were caused by cancer, but he wasn't really sure what was causing them, and I think he didn't want to contradict the oncologist. In the meantime, I went to a dermatologist for a red rash that I had on my stomach. He didn't know what the cause was and couldn't treat it. I then went to a rheumatologist; he ran all his tests and

> *While the doctors were still arguing, my family was sure that I wasn't going to live to the end of the year. I was still going for tests twice a week and giving eight or nine blood samples.*
>
> —EUGENE

again came up without a diagnosis. I know lupus is hard to diagnose, but with all the major common symptoms I had, I still can't believe someone along the line didn't put it all together sooner.

"Finally I went to a kidney specialist because my kidneys were starting to fail. The tests he ran showed that my kidneys were in really bad shape, so he said he needed a few days to carefully go over all my records and test results. After about three days he called and said, 'I'm about 95 percent sure what's wrong with you. I think it's lupus, but I want to do a kidney biopsy to confirm the diagnosis.' Sure enough, he was right. After 2 years, 2 months, and 19 doctors, I finally had a name for my illness. I didn't know what lupus was, but at least it was a definite diagnosis.

"This doctor immediately started treating my kidneys with medication and I've been doing very well for quite a while now. Getting this diagnosis put me through the worst 2 years of my life. I'm hoping that my story will help other people and maybe they won't have to go through what I went through." Let us hope that Eugene is right. As more people understand the complicated and often confusing symptoms of lupus, more will proactively ask for lupus testing.

> *After 2 years, 2 months, and 19 doctors, I finally had a name for my illness. I didn't know what lupus was, but at least it was a definite diagnosis.*
>
> —EUGENE

Although Eugene's story sadly isn't unique, the search for a diagnosis doesn't have to be like this. With the right doctor, the process can be much simpler. Consider Tiffany, whom you met in chapter 1, whose lupus symptoms first flared after her father's sudden death. She went to a doctor in June and was diagnosed with lupus by July. There are physicians out there who know how to recognize the deceptive symptoms of lupus. The key is to find them.

FINDING THE RIGHT DOCTOR

The typical search for a diagnosis often begins with your general practitioner, who will (or should) begin with a thorough medical history, a physical exam, and diagnostic laboratory tests. This information will help your doctor determine if your symptoms and signs of disease fit the standard criteria established for diagnosing lupus. If your symptoms or blood tests indicate possible lupus, your primary care physician should refer you to a specialist, probably a rheumatologist. You can and should take an active role in finding the specialist who is right for you.

Gloria Spadaro, R.N., executive director of the New Jersey chapter of the Lupus Foundation of America, often advises people how to find the right doctor. "If you have kidney problems," she says, "you might be seeing a nephrologist, or if you have problems with your blood, you might be seeing a hematologist, and so on. But if you don't yet have a diagnosis of lupus and you suspect something more is going on, you should see a rheumatologist; that's generally the person who has knowledge of the total picture of lupus. Representatives from any Lupus Foundation of America branch can give you a list of rheumatologists who can diagnose and treat lupus. Or, if you have access to a computer, you can go to the Web site of the American College of Rheumatology (ACR) at www.rheumatology.org and click on the link "Find a Rheumatologist" and get a whole list of doctors in your state. (Keep in mind that only those physicians who are members of ACR are listed; this doesn't mean there aren't other qualified physicians in your area as well.) Then, if you have an HMO insurance policy, you will narrow down the list by identifying the ones who participate in your health plan."

Once you have this list, your real work of finding the right physician begins. "Just because a physician is on a list provided by the Lupus Foundation or the College of Rheumatology," says Spadaro, "doesn't mean he or she is the right one for you. These organizations can't recommend anyone; they can only give you access to choices. To be honest, there are some doctors on our list that I wouldn't go to, but I can't deny people access to them. And sometimes you'll find that some rheumatologists specialize in only arthritis or only gerontology and so on. So it's not a bad idea to call and ask if the doctor treats

Speaking Out

The following quotes are from online message boards that are found on various lupus Web sites where people can share their thoughts, questions, and concerns:

"The doctor has finally decided to refer to what I have as 'lupus.' Why are they so afraid to use that word?"

"Had a miserable trip to the hospital for a test yesterday. I was proclaimed normal and officially off-my-rocker."

"I know how awful it is to have tests run only for them to say everything looks normal or misdiagnose you altogether. You know when your body isn't right and you just need to keep pushing! That's what I did and hopefully I will be seeing results soon. (I hope!) Don't let them get you down because that's not going to help you."

"My primary doc is 'overwhelmed' by all my tests, doctors, etc., and said she would scream if she were handed one more paper. I asked about my test results and it turns out that the nurse didn't put the blood in the right tube and it could not be tested . . . but

lupus patients and then schedule a visit to see if you like the doctor and feel he or she is competent."

Spadaro knows from personal experience how difficult it can be to find the right physician to treat lupus. She herself was diagnosed 26 years ago, but 15 years prior to that she was misdiagnosed over and over. "I remember complaining of joint pains in high school and being told they were growing pains and I'd get over it. Then I went to a skin doctor for 3 years for a rash that I'd get every time I went out in the sun. Then I went to Florida and the strong sun there triggered more symptoms, but it still took from July to the following May to get the correct diagnosis. In that time, I had a sore throat and was the doc doesn't want to redraw blood for that right now because she is too 'overwhelmed.' How drawing blood is that much of a strain on her, I will never know."

"I have a friend who has asked me for some help. She has been to a rheumatologist who just said that she is depressed, prescribed her some antidepression drug, and sent her on her way. She has the extreme fatigue, numbness, and tingling in her extremities, malaise, skin rashes on the neck and face, weight loss, sensitivity to sunlight, severe joint and muscle pain, nausea, severe chest pain and trouble breathing, and visual blurring to name a few. She is desperate for answers and seeks a good physician."

"After reading so many posts about really bad doctors, I feel I should count my blessings, again, for I love my rheumatologist! She's a woman, she's a minority, and she's a healthy size, so she breaks a lot of molds! I've been with her now for about 3 years, and I actually look forward to seeing her! Keep hope, those of you who haven't found your 'prince (or princess!) charming' of doctors—there are some good ones out there!!"

treated with penicillin, which really made the symptoms of lupus blossom. I still don't have a positive blood test all the time. If I'm given estrogen, or something else that brings it out, then I test positive, but not all the time.

"It's very difficult for most of us, but things are changing in the doctor-patient relationship that we should take advantage of. When I was a young nurse, when the doctor walked into the nurses' station, you stood up to greet him. It's not that way anymore. You have the right to ask questions and get understandable answers. Remember, when you're looking for a doctor, you are a consumer buying a service. If you find you don't like the way the service is provided, you should let the doctor know your concerns and, if not satisfied with the explanations, you should look for another physician."

Michael Gross, M.D., associate professor at New York University Medical Center, is a rheumatologist who treats lupus patients and who agrees that it can take time and effort to find the right doctor. "This is a complicated disease and you need a doctor with the kind of experience necessary to treat it. A doctor may have a few mild-lupus patients in his practice, but if that doctor hasn't spent time with sick lupus patients in the hospital, he may not be the one to help you when you need it most. You also don't want a physician who was trained 25 years ago and has not kept up on lupus management."

> *You have the right to ask questions and get understandable answers. When you're looking for a doctor, you are a consumer buying a service.*
>
> —GLORIA SPADARO, R.N.

So, when you're looking for a doctor, how can you know if the doctor is trained and experienced? Dr. Gross says you might try to find out before making an appointment by calling the office and asking how many lupus patients the doctor has and when and where the doctor trained in lupus. "Unfortunately," admits Dr. Gross, "you might not get complete or accurate answers to these questions from the receptionist and it's unlikely that the doctor will come to the phone to verify his background. You can also find doctors who are involved with lupus by reading medical literature and seeing if any physicians in your area are publishing on this subject. Also, you can find out which physicians are on the board of local lupus organizations or at least are on the referral list of these organizations. You might also call the office on joint disease at a medical or academic center in a major city near you and ask for a referral to physicians who have trained in their facilities and who now practice in your area."

IT TAKES TEAMWORK

Once you find a physician who can diagnose and treat lupus, it is then important to make sure that this is a person who is willing to develop a team relationship built on mutual respect. Dr. Gross believes that a good doctor-patient relationship requires effort on the part of both the patient and the doctor.

In detailing the patient's responsibilities, Dr. Gross says, "Patients need to be involved in their own care. They should keep a timeline of their symptoms, so they can accurately report when certain things happened and under what conditions. I think patients also have a responsibility to be compliant with the doctor's instructions. They have to keep their medical appointments and keep track of their medications and take them when they're supposed to. They also need to have an appreciation of what is and what is not worth worrying about. They can't arrive at the doctor's office with a list of 25 things that they are overly anxious about and expect the doctor to have time to discuss and analyze every one. At the same time, they shouldn't withhold information that could be important."

> *Once you find a physician who can diagnose and treat lupus, it is then important to make sure that this is a person who is willing to develop a team relationship built on mutual respect.*

Dr. Gross believes that you can learn how to find the line between what's important to bring to your doctor's attention and what's not by making an effort to become educated about lupus. "There's a lot of misinformation out there," he admits, "but if you stick to literature and Internet sites that are reputable, like those of the Lupus Foundation and the National Institutes of Health, you can find out a lot about your disease. By being educated, you can ask your doctor direct and important questions that don't waste time, but still give you the personalized information you need."

Dr. Gross is quick to point out that the doctor, too, has responsibilities in this relationship. "The doctor should give patients a sense of confidence in his ability to understand and treat the disease," he says. "He should give the patient educational materials to answer basic questions and he should be honest about what could happen if the disease progresses. He should be clear about what symptoms to watch for and explain that, although the symptoms might be quite mild at that time, the disease might progress and what might happen if it does. Doctors also need to be accessible. If the doctor has 350 patients, it's very easy to get lost. The fact is that some rheumatologists may not want to care for sick lupus patients because it can be very, very time-consuming. That's why you should look for a doctor who has an interest in treating lupus patients and, at the same time, has a lot of experience with this disease. I think this is even more important than personality."

All of this searching does take time, but with a chronic illness like lupus, you're building a long-term relationship, so you have many valid reasons to make sure it will be a good one.

A Good Match

Dr. Gross has a loyal following of patients who respect him for both his sense of compassion and his dedication to treating this difficult disease. Donna, 53, a former nurse who is now on permanent disability, is one of them. "I love my doctor," she says. "He is not only understanding, but is also a strong advocate for lupus patients. This past spring I was invited to go to Washington to explain to Congress how lupus has affected my life. When I told Dr. Gross about it, he asked if he could go, too. It turned out that I had to go into the hospital for lupus complications, so I couldn't go to Washington, but Dr. Gross went, and took my letter along with 26 others I had collected from other lupus patients telling how lupus affects them. He made copies of all our letters, and he handed them to everyone he met. He personally made sure our stories would be heard. He is now active in our local Lupus Foundation of America group, and has recently been elected to our board of directors."

Donna knows that all lupus patients are not as lucky. "I belong to an online lupus group," she says, "and the biggest complaint I hear is

> *Some rheumatologists may not want to care for sick lupus patients because it can be very, very time-consuming. That's why you should look for a doctor who has an interest in treating lupus patients and, at the same time, has a lot of experience with this disease.*

about doctors. I know it's very hard to diagnose and treat lupus because it mimics so many other diseases, so a lot of people go undiagnosed or receive inadequate care for years. I feel so bad for them. I have been fortunate; I receive excellent care from my group of lupus physicians. Having a nursing background, I have met many, many doctors, but from the first time I met Dr. Gross, he stood out. His sincere concern and compassion for the lupus patient shows in his dedication. Other doctors tend to talk *at* you; he listens! I can talk to Dr. Gross and know that he is 'hearing' me. He sits down, makes direct eye contact, and doesn't interrupt. This makes me feel like I can be open and honest with him, which makes for a good patient-doctor relationship. He realizes that this disease affects all parts of our lives, not just what's written in my chart. I know I'm not just a lupus patient to him; I'm a person with a disease called lupus. . . . There is a difference."

Time for a Second Opinion

It's time to get a second opinion or find a new doctor if you believe that you have the classic symptoms of lupus, and:

- Your doctor orders dozens of tests and then decides "there's nothing wrong with you."

- You explain your concern about possible lupus and your doctor doesn't seem interested in discussing the possibility.

- Your primary care doctor won't give you a referral to a specialist.

- Your doctor regards your symptoms as signs of stress or depression.

- Your doctor doesn't have time to listen to you because each patient visit is limited to a certain number of minutes.

Help Yourself

Once you find a doctor you like, you should make the effort to be proactive in your own care. Your doctor needs to know everything about your health in order to know if you meet the diagnostic criteria for lupus established by the American College of Rheumatology. Here are some things you can do to help your doctor correctly diagnosis your illness:

- If you have a skin rash that comes and goes, take a picture of it, so the doctor can see what it looks like if the rash should disappear the day of your appointment.

- Go to your medical appointment prepared with written information. Write down:

    1. All your symptoms.
    2. All the doctors you've seen in your search for a diagnosis and provide their addresses and phone numbers.
    3. Results of all diagnostic tests you've taken so far; this gives the doctor necessary background information and will also help avoid unnecessary repetition of tests.
    4. All medications you take (prescription and over-the-counter drugs).

- Be thorough and honest. When you have the opportunity to talk to the doctor, don't hide or forget any medical information. If, for example, out of embarrassment, people neglect to mention positive syphilis test results, they withhold an important piece of information that could lead to a more rapid diagnosis (because people with lupus frequently have a false-positive syphilis test).

STANDARD CRITERIA FOR DIAGNOSING LUPUS

In 1971, to help researchers identify people with systemic lupus erythematosus in epidemiologic studies, the American College of Rheumatology devised criteria for defining the disease. These criteria were revised in 1982 and again in 1996.[1] This standard identification tool states that the diagnosis of lupus can be confirmed when a patient presents with at least four of 11 criteria. It must be noted that these criteria are helpful in differentiating SLE from disorders such as rheumatoid arthritis. Rheumatologists do not make the diagnosis of lupus by strictly adhering to these criteria, however, but may base the diagnosis on fewer than four of these signs combined with other signs such as fever, hair loss, stroke, pneumonitis, or nerve damage. The ACR criteria are helpful, though, in identifying many of the characteristic signs of lupus.

The first four criteria focus on symptoms related to the skin:

1. Rash over the cheeks: the characteristic butterfly rash.

2. Discoid rash: raised red patches that cause scars and appear usually on sun-exposed areas.

3. Photosensitivity: rash after being exposed to ultraviolet A and B light.

4. Ulcers in the mouth or nose: usually painless and recurrent.

The next four ACR criteria focus on specific organ areas:

5. Arthritis: non-erosive arthritis in which the bones around the joints do not become destroyed; inflammation of two peripheral joints with tenderness, swelling, or fluid.

6. Pleuritis or pericarditis: inflammation of the lining of the lung or heart.

7. Kidney disorder: excessive protein or abnormal sediment in the urine.

8. Neurologic disorder: seizures, convulsions, or psychosis with no other explanation.

The final three criteria specify laboratory abnormalities of the disease:

9.   Blood abnormalities: hemolytic anemia, low white blood cell counts, low platelet counts.

10. Positive antinuclear antibody (ANA) test.

11. Immunologic disorder: antibodies to Sm nuclear antigen, antibodies to native DNA, or positive results of antiphospholipid antibodies test based on an abnormal serum level of IgG or IgM anticardiolipin antibodies, a positive test result for lupus anticoagulant, or a false-positive serologic test for syphilis known to be positive for at least 6 months.

Remember, you won't have all of these symptoms and you might not have the symptoms all the time or even at the same time. Your specific diagnosis may be based on these or other criteria.

LABORATORY TESTS

If you have lupus, you have an autoimmune disorder in which the immune system loses its ability to tell the difference between foreign substances and its own cells and tissues. As explained in chapter 1, the immune system then makes antibodies directed against the body's healthy cells and tissues. These antibodies, called autoantibodies,

---

Lupus Diagnosis

Lupus is a multi-symptom disease. To diagnose, physicians typically look for abnormalities in one or more of the following:

Blood	Lungs
Heart	Nervous system
Joints	Skin
Kidney	

"attack" various parts of the body, causing inflammation, injury to tissues, and pain. Several diagnostic blood tests look for these autoantibodies and measure the activity (or overactivity) of the immune system. Other tests assess the health of specific organs such as the kidneys.

Tests commonly used in the diagnosis of SLE are the following.

Antinuclear antibody test (ANA). To determine if autoantibodies to cell nuclei are present in the blood.

Anti-DNA antibody test. To determine if the patient has antibodies to the main genetic material in the nucleus of the cell.

Anti-Sm antibody test. To determine if there are antibodies to Sm, which is a protein found in the cell nucleus.

Blood complement level test. To examine the total level of serum complement, a group of proteins involved in the inflammation in immune reactions, and to assess the specific level of C3 and C4, two proteins of this group.

Tissue biopsy. To examine the type and extent of tissue damage or inflammation and its cause.

Let's look at each of these tests more closely.

Antinuclear Antibody Test (ANA)

The antinuclear antibody test determines if autoantibodies to the nucleus of the cell are present in the blood. It is also sometimes called the fluorescent antinuclear antibody test or FANA. Over 90 percent of people with lupus will have a positive reaction to this test, particularly when they have active disease. This makes it the best and most sensitive diagnostic test currently available for identifying systemic lupus.

A negative ANA test result is strong evidence against lupus as the cause of illness, but there are infrequent instances where SLE is present without detectable antinuclear antibodies. Naturally, this possibility is frustrating for those who receive a negative result and are misled into thinking that, although they have some of the symptoms of lupus, they couldn't possibly have the disease. As one young woman posted on a lupus message board: "It was really nice when my doctor said he thought I had lupus. For a couple of days I thought there was a logical reason behind what I've been going through, but now that my ANA came back negative, I'm back to square one." If you are experiencing the symptoms of lupus but have a negative ANA, your doctor will probably test you for other autoantibodies (as explained later in this chapter) that can also indicate lupus.

A negative ANA test result is strong evidence against lupus as the cause of illness, but there are infrequent instances where SLE is present without detectable antinuclear antibodies.

A positive ANA test result will help a physician diagnose lupus, but a positive result by itself is not proof of lupus because the test may also be positive in numerous other conditions, including:

- Other autoimmune and connective tissue diseases such as rheumatoid arthritis, scleroderma, Sjögren's syndrome, and Hashimoto's thyroiditis.

- Liver disease, infectious mononucleosis, and chronic infectious diseases such as hepatitis, lepromatous leprosy, subacute bacterial endocarditis, and malaria.

- When patients are being treated with certain drugs, such as procainamide, hydralazine, isoniazid, or chlorpromazine.

Interestingly, the test can also be weakly positive in about 20 percent of healthy individuals. The "weak" or "strong" degree of an ANA test result is determined by the titer that accompanies the report. The titer is a number that indicates how many times the technician had to dilute plasma from the person's blood to get a sample free of the antinuclear antibodies. For example, a titer of 1:80 means the technician had to dilute the sample 80 times. A titer above 1:80 is usually considered positive, but obviously a titer of 1:320 shows a greater concentration of antinuclear antibodies and thus a "stronger" positive test result.

The microscopic blood pattern of the ANA test result can be used to separate the likelihood of lupus from other autoimmune diseases. Results appear in a smooth (or diffuse), speckled, or rimmed peripheral pattern. The smooth pattern is found in a variety of connective tissue diseases as well as in patients taking particular drugs such as certain antiarrhythmics, anticonvulsants, or antihypertensives. This nonspecific pattern is also the one that is most commonly seen in healthy individuals who have a positive ANA test. The speckled pattern is found in SLE and other connective tissue diseases, while the peripheral (or rim) pattern is found primarily in patients who have lupus with organ disease such as nephritis.

Remember that the diagnosis is a clinical one, which means that it is *supported* but not made or confirmed by a blood test. In putting the results together, however, if your ANA test comes back positive with a high titer and a speckled or peripheral pattern, your physician will feel more confident in an accurate diagnosis of lupus than if your results come back positive, but with a low titer and a smooth pattern. In either case, if you have other symptoms or signs of lupus, your physician will probably want to conduct further tests for lupus or refer you at that time to a specialist to continue the testing.

> *R*emember that the diagnosis is a clinical one, which means that it is supported *but not made or confirmed by a blood test.*

Anti-DNA Antibody Test

Deoxyribonucleic acid (DNA, the chemical in the cell nuclei that makes up the body's genetic code) is fundamental to life. The body does not normally make antibodies directed against it—unless a person has an autoimmune disease. Antibodies to double-stranded DNA are found specifically in lupus and are detected through the anti-native DS (double-stranded) DNA antibody test.

Anti-Sm Antibody Test

"Sm" is short for "Smith," the person in which this particular protein was first found. Antibodies to the Sm antigen are found almost exclusively in lupus and are present in 30 to 40 percent of lupus cases.[2] A positive test result generally means that the person has lupus; false positives are rare. A negative result, however, does not mean that lupus is not present. Other tests can still be positive. Most people with lupus have either anti-DNA or anti-Sm antibodies. Negative tests for both generally mean that lupus is not present.[3]

Blood Complement Level Test

Complement is a blood protein that destroys bacteria and also causes inflammation. Complement proteins are identified by the letter C and a number. The most common complement tests for lupus are C3, C4, and CH50. If the total blood complement level is low (because the immune reaction consumes complement components), or the C3 or C4 complement values are low and there is also a positive ANA, the possibility of lupus increases. Low C3 and C4 complement levels in people with positive ANA and anti-DNA tests may indicate active lupus kidney disease.

Tissue Biopsy

A tissue biopsy is one of the best ways to examine a tissue or organ sample when testing for lupus. This procedure involves removing a small sliver of tissue, which is then examined under a microscope. When a skin rash is present and the cause is unknown, a biopsy can be helpful. A lupus rash will show a characteristic deposit of antibody and complement in the upper border of the skin. A kidney biopsy may be needed to better define the type and extent of kidney involvement. A kidney biopsy may show deposits of antibodies, immune complexes, and complement as well as specific patterns of inflammation that can guide therapy and help with prognosis.

Other Diagnostic Tests

There are many other tests that can be used to help put all the lupus puzzle pieces together. Their names tend to become a jumble of letters, but the following descriptions will give you some idea of the testing your doctor is prescribing.

Complete Blood Count (CBC)

This test includes the following.

Hemoglobin and hematocrit. Low levels define anemia due to immunologic damage or active inflammation.

White blood cell count and differential count. Low levels can reflect immunologic damage, active lupus, and increased risk for infection.

Platelet count. Low levels reflect immunologic damage and may lead to bleeding.

Erythrocyte Sedimentation Rate (Sed Rate or ESR)

Elevated levels reflect the state of inflammation or the presence of infection.

Creactive Protein

Elevated levels reflect the state of inflammation or the presence of infection.

Kidney Tests

These tests include the following.

Serum creatinine. Elevated levels often reflect poor kidney function.

Blood urea nitrogen (BUN). Elevated levels can reflect poor kidney function, dehydration, or the effects of steroids.

Urinalysis. A microscopic test that can demonstrate active kidney inflammation and excessive excretion of protein.

24-hour protein and creatinine clearance. This 24-hour urine collection gives the most accurate measure of kidney function and protein excretion.

Antibody Tests

Your doctor will probably also want to see the results of any number of antibody tests, including any or all of the following.

Coagulation tests. Including the activated partial thromboplastic time (aPTT) test and the dilute Russell viper venom time (dRVVT) test; the times measured in these tests may be prolonged in people with the antiphospholipid antibody syndrome.

Rheumatoid factor (RF) antibody test. To distinguish lupus from rheumatoid arthritis.

Anticardiolipin (ACL) antibody test. To measure antibodies to the cardiolipin molecule (a molecule associated with phospholipid membranes in human cells and the membranes of certain bacteria; three kinds of anticardiolipin antibodies are possible: IgG, IgM, and IgA).

Other antibody tests. Many other possible tests include: antisribonucleoprotein (RNP), anti-Sjögren's syndrome A (Ro/SSA), and anti-Sjögren's syndrome B (La/SSB).

Diagnostic Procedures

Sometimes lupus is diagnosed by examining the tissue or cell damage in body organs caused by the disease. If you have lung disease, for example, your physician may order a chest x ray or a CT scan (allowing a sectional view of the body constructed by computed tomography). If you have cardiovascular problems, the doctor may want to see the results of an electrocardiogram (ECG, a recording of the changes of electrical potential occurring during the heartbeat) or echocardiogram, which uses ultrasound to examine and measure structure and functioning of the heart. Patients with central nervous system involvement may need an electroencephalogram (EEG, to detect and record brain waves), magnetic resonance imaging (MRI, a noninvasive diagnostic technique that produces computerized images of internal body tissues and is based on nuclear magnetic resonance of atoms within the body induced by the application of radio waves), or positron emission tomography (PET, noninvasive cross-sectional imaging of regional metabolism obtained by a color-coded representation of the distribution of gamma radiation given off in the collision of electrons in cells).

Sometimes Positive, Sometimes Negative

It would help doctors and their patients to better diagnose lupus if testing laboratories would standardize their procedures. Because different laboratories perform the same tests differently, it is not unusual (but very confusing) when one doctor orders a test from one laboratory that comes up positive and another doctor later orders that same test from a different laboratory and the result is then negative. The come-and-go nature of lupus further clouds the issue because some test results can change from time to time depending on the state of your health or the medications you are taking. For these reasons, your doctors may repeat tests at different times in the course of your care.

Three Factors of Diagnosis

The diagnosis of lupus is made by combining the results of these three factors:

1. Your entire medical history.

2. Your current symptoms (facts you tell the doctor) and signs (information gathered by your doctor from the physical examination and tests).

3. An analysis of the results of your laboratory tests.

THE GREAT IMPERSONATOR

The diagnosis of lupus is further complicated because there are other illnesses that have similar symptoms. Often a physician will want to rule out these possibilities before confirming lupus. There are several broad categories of lupus-like disorders that need to be ruled out during the diagnosis process. In *The Lupus Book*, Dr. Wallace describes these five.

Hormonal imbalance. Hormonal changes caused by pregnancy, thyroid abnormalities, menopause, or other factor can produce symptoms such as fatigue, aching, and fever.

Blood or tissue malignancies. These cancers, ranging from lymphoma to breast cancer, can result in positive ANAs and symptoms similar to lupus.

Infectious processes. Viruses especially are associated with positive ANAs as well as lupus-like symptoms.

Neurologic disorders. Disease states such as multiple sclerosis or myasthenia gravis can coexist with or be difficult to differentiate from SLE.

Rheumatic diseases. Especially during the first year of symptoms, rheumatoid arthritis, scleroderma, mixed connective tissue disease, inflammatory myositis, and other forms of systemic vasculitis can be very difficult to distinguish from each other and from SLE.[4]

Two specific illness that are often confused with lupus are undifferentiated connective tissue disease and Sjögren's syndrome.

Undifferentiated connective tissue disease (UCTD). An illness that can be called "almost lupus." A person with UCTD has some or many of the symptoms associated with lupus, but does not have "at least four" of the 11 standard criteria symptoms required by the American College of Rheumatology for a diagnosis of lupus. Dr. Wallace says, "There are probably a million Americans with UCTD. Its features include rashes, swollen joints, fatigue, fevers, swollen glands, Raynaud's, pleurisy, high sedimentation rates, and a positive ANA."[5] One major difference, however, is the fact that UCTD is rarely organ threatening and is less serious than SLE.

Sjögren's syndrome. Sometimes confused with lupus because they share some clinical similarities. Both are primarily found in women; both can cause joint pain; both show similar positive antibody tests; both can cause fatigue and mouth ulcers; and both respond to corticosteroid treatment. Because the two sometimes go hand in hand, it has been called the "sister disease" of lupus; however, Sjögren's syndrome is certainly not the same as lupus.[6] Sjögren's is an autoimmune disease affecting glands such as the salivary and tear glands, resulting in a lack of tears, saliva, and other glandular secretions. Ten percent of people with lupus also have obvious Sjögren's. If minimally or asymptomatic patients with lupus underwent vigorous testing for the syndrome, perhaps as many as one-third would fulfill accepted Sjögren's definitions.[7]

Because lupus can so easily be misdiagnosed and confused with other illnesses, don't be shy to ask how your doctor arrived at the diagnosis. Your doctor should be able to say something like, "Here are the published, standard criteria, and here's where you fall within that spectrum. Here are the blood test results and here is why they support the clinical diagnosis of lupus." If the doctor says you have lupus simply because everything else has been ruled out and that's what's left, ask for a second opinion.

> *If the doctor says you have lupus simply because everything else has been ruled out and that's what's left, ask for a second opinion.*

Do not let a diagnosis of lupus cause you to lump all symptoms into this one basket and chalk off all future aches and pains as lupus related. If you have other conditions commonly found in people with lupus, such as rheumatoid arthritis, Sjögren's syndrome, or Raynaud's disease, these problems must be treated separately. They cannot be lumped into the lupus pile and ignored.

If you feel any new discomfort or pain that is chronic but different from what you normally associate with lupus symptoms, don't assume it isn't anything new. Even people with lupus get kidney stones, pneumonia, and cancer. Ask yourself, "Would I go to the doctor for this pain if I did not have lupus?" If the answer is yes, then call your doctor. If your doctor should imply that you call too often, then it's time to find a new doctor.

A LONG AND PRODUCTIVE LIFE

The diagnosis of lupus brings with it mixed feelings. Many people say they feel relief to finally have a name to attach to their symptoms. They're glad to know they're not crazy or dying. They're anxious to begin treatment and get back to feeling healthy again. Mixed with the relief, many feel anxiety. It's difficult to accept the idea of a chronic disease, and worst-case scenarios are very frightening. But you must keep in mind that lupus is no longer a death sentence, especially with early diagnosis and treatment. By seeking a diagnosis, you are taking the first step toward learning how to live a long and productive life with this chronic disease. Chapter 3, "Medical Treatment," will help you take the next step toward appropriate treatment.

Medical Treatment

‹℘›

I T I S A positive sign that there have been advances in the treatment of lupus over the last few years. But at this time there is still no cure for lupus. There is no one medication or therapy that will make it go away. The best modern medicine can do is to treat the symptoms and try to prevent severe organ damage. But even this second-best approach is complex. Because lupus can affect so many different organs and systems of your body, there is no such thing as "the" treatment. Your treatment regimen must be individualized for you by your physician based on your specific symptoms and needs. And because the course of this disease changes over time, the treatment plan needs to be constantly evaluated and updated. That's why ongoing medical supervision and close partnership are absolutely essential to the effective management of lupus.

The primary treatment regimens discussed in this chapter are medications and the management of skin problems associated with lupus. Keep in mind as you read this chapter that this is a general overview of common practices. Your case and your treatment plan are individual and unique based on what you and your doctor find most effective for you.

MEDICATIONS FOR THE TREATMENT OF LUPUS

Medication as the primary method of treatment for lupus has two basic goals: to reduce the inflammation (and thus the pain) in the affected tissues and to suppress abnormalities of the immune system that may be causing the tissue inflammation and damage.[1] As the manifestations of lupus vary from person to person, however, it is often difficult to find just the right medication. The drugs used to treat lupus run the gamut from aspirin and other anti-inflammatory drugs to powerful anticancer drugs that suppress the immune system. The correct drug or combination of drugs for you depends on many factors such as medical history, the systems and symptoms involved, and the severity of the disease.

To further complicate the process of selecting the right medication, each medication has its own set of side effects that make the drug intolerable for some but don't bother others at all. It may take time, some trial and error, and patience to find the medication regimen that's best for you. Be sure to keep in close touch with your physician to let him or her know exactly how your body and your disease are reacting to any prescribed medication.

With so many drugs to choose from, it's ironic that most drugs used in the treatment of lupus are not approved by the FDA (Food and Drug Administration) specifically for this purpose. Doctors use what's called "off label" prescribing (using medications approved for other medical conditions) to help their lupus patients live better with this disease. The drugs accepted as standard practice in the treatment of this disease include:

- Nonsteroidal anti-inflammatory drugs (NSAIDs)
- Steroids
- Antimalarial drugs
- Immunosuppressive drugs

Following is an overview of each one that will give you the basic knowledge you need to better understand your treatment plan.

All Drugs Have Three Names

Every drug has a chemical name that is generally not well known except to chemists working in the laboratory. Every drug also has a generic name, which is a shortened version of the complicated chemical name; this name is used to refer to the drug regardless of manufacturer and is not capitalized the way trade names are. The third name is the trade name, which is the name the manufacturer uses to identify its product; trade names are capitalized.

You should know both the generic and trade names for every medication you take, so when you read about a drug or your doctor talks about your medication, you won't be confused by the interchangeable names.

Nonsteroidal Anti-Inflammatory Drugs

As the name indicates, nonsteroidal anti-inflammatory drugs (NSAIDs) reduce inflammation without the use of steroids. There are at least 20 different types of NSAIDs on the market today that are commonly prescribed to relieve the lupus symptoms caused by inflammation, which manifests as joint swelling, stiffness, and pain, muscle aches, or pleurisy.

NSAIDs work mainly by preventing the formation of prostaglandins (via their inhibition of enzymes called COX-1 and COX-2). These are natural substances produced by the body that play a role in causing inflammation and pain. By inhibiting their production, the inflammatory and pain process is reduced.

Some NSAIDs are available over the counter without a prescription; most require a doctor's prescription. All of the commonly available NSAIDs listed in table 1, except for celecoxib and rofecoxib, inhibit both COX-1 and COX-2 enzymes and are called traditional

Table 1.   Nonsteroidal Anti-Inflammatory Drugs (NSAIDs)

Generic Name	Trade Name(s)
celecoxib	Celebrex
diclofenac	Voltaren, Cataflam
diflunisal	Dolobid
etodolac	Lodine
fenoprofen	Nalfon
flurbiprofen	Ansaid
ibuprofen	Motrin, Advil
indomethacin	Indocin
ketoprofen	Orudis, Oruvail
ketorolac	Toradol
magnesium salicylate	Magan, Doan's
meclofenamates	Meclomen, Ponstel
meloxican	Mobic
nabumetone	Relafen
naproxen	Naprosyn, Anaprox, Aleve
oxaprozin	Daypro
piroxicam	Feldene
rofecoxib	Vioxx
sodium salicylates	Trilisate, Disalcid
sulindac	Clinoril
tolmetin sodium	Tolectin

NSAIDs. The other two NSAIDs are called COX-2 specific NSAIDs because they inhibit only the COX-2 enzyme, thus leading to fewer gastrointestinal problems and no platelet inhibition. Acetylsalicylic acid (aspirin) is also an anti-inflammatory when given in high doses; otherwise it is just a painkiller like acetaminophen (Tylenol).

You may respond better to one NSAID than to another, so it may be necessary to try a brief 3-week course of several different kinds before you find the one most effective for you. When searching for the "right one," remember that although most NSAIDs work fairly rapidly, it may take 3 or 4 weeks before you experience the full benefit.

If well tolerated, NSAIDs can be effective as the only treatment necessary for people with mild lupus localized to the joints. They can be used in combination with stronger medications to treat greater disease activity in joints and the pleura. They are not effective in serious cases with organ inflammation (such as kidney or brain involvement) and may actually worsen kidney disease.

Side Effects of NSAIDs

As with all medications, you may or may not experience adverse reactions when taking NSAIDs. In their article, "Nonsteroidal Anti-Inflammatory Drugs," Drs. Cynthia Aranow and Arthur Weinstein of New York Medical College remind us that, "While NSAIDs are widely used with good results and without problems, individuals with lupus and their prescribing doctors need to pay special attention to the potential side effects. Since drug side effects and symptoms of increased lupus activity may be identical, it is important to alert a physician if any of these symptoms occur."[2] Drs. Aranow and Weinstein describe possible side effects as follows:

Stomach upset. NSAIDs may cause dyspepsia, a burning, bloated feeling in the pit of the stomach. This happens because, in addition to inhibiting the prostaglandins that cause inflammation and pain, traditional NSAIDs (but not the COX-2 specific NSAIDs) also inhibit the prostaglandins that protect the lining of the stomach. In some cases, this lack of protection results in stomach inflammation (gastritis) or gastric ulcers. This can cause bleeding (either obvious and painful or hidden and painless) that can lead to anemia.

To help protect the stomach, you should always take NSAIDs with food or directly after a meal. Some people may need additional medications such as antacids, H-2 blockers such as ranitidine (Zantac), Cytotec, or an acid pump inhibitor such as Prilosec to control their stomach symptoms. In high-risk patients, which includes those with a history of stomach problems, the elderly, and those also on steroids, COX-2 specific NSAIDs are safer for the stomach. If you take NSAIDs for a long period of time, you should have a blood count periodically to ensure that anemia from gastric bleeding is not occurring. Also, before taking NSAIDs, be sure to tell your doctor if you have a history of gastric (stomach) or duodenal (intestinal) ulcers.

Blood abnormalities. Traditional NSAIDs (not COX-2 specific ones) affect the function of blood platelets. This is a type of blood cell important in normal blood clotting. Although aspirin has the greatest effect, all traditional NSAIDs have some effect on platelet function. If the function of these cells is impaired, it will take longer for blood to clot, and bruising can occur more readily. Some people are especially vulnerable to this side effect and may need to discontinue the medication. All of these medications should be stopped in those who develop thrombocytopenia (low platelets) or who are going to have surgery.

Kidney and blood pressure effects. NSAIDs can cause fluid retention, high blood pressure, and reduced kidney function in people who have lupus-related kidney or blood pressure problems. Because NSAIDs can cause further deterioration in kidney function, people with lupus nephritis, who already have reduced kidney function, should avoid taking them.

Rare side effects. Several rare side effects of NSAIDs can be mistaken for signs of lupus. The drugs may cause fever or skin rashes that can easily be confused with signs of active lupus. The drugs may produce changes in the kidney leading to edema or abnormalities on uri-nalysis or blood tests that resemble lupus nephritis. Similarly, certain nonsteroidal drugs have been shown to cause fever and headache that can mimic a type of meningitis seen in lupus.

It's important to recognize all of the above side effects promptly. Too often people suffer with headaches, rashes, and the like, thinking they're inevitable symptoms of lupus, when in fact they're side effects of NSAIDs that can be reversed simply by stopping the drug. If you are taking NSAIDs daily for long-term treatment, be sure to have complete blood work done, along with liver and kidney blood chemistries, and blood pressure monitoring at least every 3 to 4 months.

Antimalarial Drugs

An antimalarial drug? Isn't that a medication to prevent and treat ma-laria? Well, yes it is, but quite by accident it was also found to be helpful to people with lupus and rheumatoid arthritis. During World War II, troops in the Pacific theater faced the serious threat of malaria and so were given antimalarial medication for 3 years. There were anecdotal reports that soldiers with arthritis or lupus experienced improvement in

---

Don't Be Afraid

"The primary treatment protocol for lupus is medications," says Jimmy Lawrence, M.D. "But unfortunately," says Dr. Lawrence, "people have become afraid of drugs and their side effects. So often I have to convince my patients that medication is necessary and good. Of course, I would do anything to avoid medications where possible, but when the benefit is so much higher than the risk, we can't be frightened to use them—with the goal of reducing the dosage and frequency over time."

rashes and joint symptoms when they took this medication. This led the British to conduct a study of the efficacy of antimalarials in treating lupus. The positive findings were published in the English journal *Lancet* in 1951 and antimalarials have been used to treat lupus ever since.[3]

Antimalarials work to relieve the symptoms of mild, non-organ threatening lupus in a variety of ways:

- They block ultraviolet light from damaging skin.
- They have an anti-inflammatory effect similar to NSAIDs, which can ease muscle and joint pain and reduce inflammation of the lining of the heart (pericarditis) and lungs (pleuritis).
- They reduce fatigue and fever.
- They are very effective in the treatment of discoid lupus erythematosus. Sixty to 90 percent of people with DLE went into remission or showed major improvement after being treated with antimalarials.
- Skin lesions of DLE that have not responded to treatment with topical therapies can improve with the use of antimalarial drugs.
- They inhibit clotting (a problem for some people with lupus).
- They help reduce mouth ulcers and hair loss.
- They can improve cognitive dysfunction.[4]

There are three antimalarials most commonly used to treat the symptoms of lupus: Plaquenil (hydroxychloroquine sulfate), Aralen (chloroquine), and Atabrine (quinacrine). Plaquenil is the only antimalarial currently both approved by the FDA and promoted specifically for lupus. It is very effective for many people.

In 1991, a group of Canadian rheumatologists studied 47 patients whose mild, non-organ threatening lupus was under good control with Plaquenil. Half of the patients received a placebo (sugar pill) and the other half continued their Plaquenil. The Plaquenil group had many fewer disease flare-ups and organ-threatening complications over a 6-month period. This study confirmed previous suggestions that the institution of antimalarial therapy early in the disease course decreases the risk that lupus will spread to critical organs.[5]

Unfortunately, Plaquenil is slow acting, and so it usually takes several months to achieve maximum benefit. On the plus side, however, if the drug is effective, you can safely take it for an extended period of time. Dr. Daniel Wallace has found that about half of his patients on Plaquenil with mild, non-organ threatening lupus are 80 to 90 percent better after 2 to 3 years. About half of them are able to discontinue the drug after 3 to 4 years.[6]

Aralen is also FDA-approved for the treatment of lupus, but because of its greater potential for eye toxicity it is not used often. Aralen is a more potent drug that is faster acting than Plaquenil and is particularly effective for skin rashes and joint inflammation.

Atabrine is a very safe and effective antimalarial drug. Due to its decreased availability, the U.S. Army has sequestered the supply in order to make it available for resistant malaria. However, it can be compounded by companies such as Panorama.

Often antimalarials are used in combination with other medications. For example, Plaquenil may be prescribed to control skin lesions while a steroid such as prednisone may be necessary to suppress the immune system and quickly reduce inflammation. Also, antimalarials can be used to enhance the positive effects and reduce the side effects of steroids. They can lower the cholesterol raised by steroids and decrease the tendency of steroids to promote clots. They can also be used to help wean an individual off steroids completely.

> *Antimalarials can be used to enhance the positive effects and reduce the side effects of steroids. They can also be used to help wean an individual off steroids completely.*

Side Effects of Antimalarial Drugs

Antimalarials are relatively mild, safe drugs and, unlike more potent drugs used to treat lupus, they do not lower blood counts or make people more susceptible to infection. But like all drugs, there are some possible side effects you should be aware of. They can cause skin rashes and pigmentary changes (particularly a yellowing of the skin with the use of quinacrine). They can also cause digestive upset such as loss of appetite, abdominal bloating, cramps, nausea, vomiting, and diarrhea. These side effects usually go away after an individual adjusts to the medication, but if they persist, you should stop taking the medication, which will stop the side effects.

A more serious side effect is the possibility that antimalarial drugs may damage the retina of the eye, resulting in visual disturbances, even blindness. It is important to note that retinal damage is dose related and the low doses used in the treatment of lupus are rarely associated with retinal damage. Most cases of eye disease occur in patients taking more than 400 milligrams of Plaquenil or more than 250 milligrams of Aralen daily.[7]

Retinal damage due to the use of Plaquenil is sometimes reversible, if it is treated early. Damage due to Aralen, however, is irreversible. That is why it is so necessary, before beginning treatment with antimalarials, to see an eye doctor or ophthalmologist for a baseline examination and to have follow-up eye examinations every 3 to 6 months thereafter. On many occasions, an ophthalmologist can see mild changes in the retinal pigment that indicate early damage due to the use of antimalarials. In addition to the regular eye checkups, which test visual acuity and eye pressure, tests of color vision and visual field might be necessary. New computer-assisted machines for testing the visual field for antimalarial effects are very sensitive to small changes. Individuals can also monitor themselves between visits by the use of something called an amsler grid, which can be obtained from an ophthalmologist. If visual symptoms do occur (blurred vision or any other changes), report them immediately to your doctor.[8]

Overall, antimalarials are safe drugs. Most patients report no side effects at all and, with patience and time, often find the drugs helpful in the management of lupus symptoms.

Steroids

When the symptoms of lupus are severe and cannot be controlled by NSAIDs or antimalarials, the physician's next line of treatment therapy may be steroids. Cortisone and its steroid derivatives are the most effective anti-inflammatory drugs known. They can substantially reduce the swelling, tenderness, pain, and internal inflammation associated with lupus.

Steroids produced by the cortex (outer portion) of the adrenal glands (see figure 3.1) are called "corticosteroids." Synthetically produced corticosteroids are extremely effective drugs that can quickly reduce inflammation and suppress activity of the immune system. They are lifesavers for many people with lupus.

The most commonly prescribed synthetic corticosteroid for the treatment of lupus is prednisone. Prednisone comes in tablets of 1, 5, 10, and 20 milligrams. Robert Katz, M.D., of the Presbyterian St. Luke Medical Center in Chicago, Illinois, says that patients can take this drug as often as four times daily, as infrequently as once every other day, or at any frequency in between. Dr. Katz says, "Less than

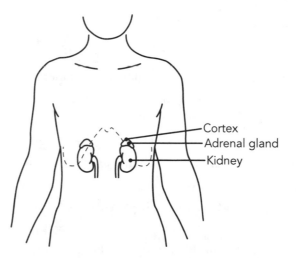

Figure 3.1—*The Adrenal Glands*

Corticosteroids

Corticosteroids commonly used in the treatment of lupus are:

- Orasone and Deltra (prednisone). Most frequently prescribed of the corticosteroids used to treat lupus.

- Hydeltra (prednisolone). Chemically changed for easy passage through the liver.

- Hydrocortone (hydrocortisone).Weaker in strength than prednisone and is more promoting of fluid and salt retention.

- Medrol (methylprednisolone). Stronger than prednisone and less promoting of fluid and salt retention.

- Decadron (dexamethasone). Extremely potent but used only in unusual circumstances because of its greater tendency for side effects.

- Topical corticosteroid cream and ointments are also available for skin problems associated with lupus (see page 91 for more details).

10 milligrams per day is generally considered a low dose; 11 to 40 milligrams daily is a moderate dose; and 41 to 100 milligrams daily is a high dose."[9] Steroids can also be given by intramuscular (IM) or intravenous (IV) injections or injected directly into a joint.

In some severe cases, when the physician feels there is danger to significant organs, you may need what's called pulse therapy (also known as *bolus* therapy). This involves intravenous administration of large amounts of corticosteroids over a short period of time, such as 3 hours during monthly 3-day therapy sessions. The effects of pulse therapy with steroids such as methylprednisolone (Medrol) often last for weeks. In order to monitor for side effects, pulse therapy usually requires a hospital stay or observation in an infusion unit.

If your doctor decides to prescribe a corticosteroid to treat your lupus, he or she will carefully individualize the type and dose based on your personal needs. If you have symptoms such as fever, arthritis, or pleurisy that have not responded to nonsteroidal anti-inflammatory drugs, you may be treated with low doses of an oral corticosteroid such as prednisone or methylprednisolone. On the other hand, if you have more severe or serious manifestations of lupus, such as nephritis, hemolytic anemia, or low platelets (thrombocytopenia), or central nervous system involvement, you may require high doses. In general, once the symptoms of lupus have responded to treatment with corticosteroids, the doctor gradually reduces the dose while carefully monitoring the patient for signs of relapse.[10]

Many people are initially very happy with the effects of corticosteroids. The drugs can dramatically ease lupus symptoms and also give a feeling of euphoria and great energy. The dosage of corticosteroids needs to be carefully regulated and monitored, however, because of the variety of side effects associated with these drugs. You and your physician may need to experiment carefully for a while to find the dose that maximizes the beneficial anti-immune and anti-inflammatory effects and minimizes the negative side effects.

Side Effects of Steroids

The use of steroids to treat lupus has been called a double-edged sword. On the one side, they save many lives. On the other side, they can cause serious complications.

Side effects of corticosteroids that Dr. Katz advises you to watch out for and talk to your doctor about the following.

Changes in physical appearance. Steroids can cause acne, a round or moon-shaped face, an increase in appetite leading to weight gain, and thinning hair. They may also cause a redistribution of fat, leading to a swollen face and abdomen, but thin arms and legs. In some cases, the skin can become more fragile, leading to easy bruising.

Mood changes. Psychological side effects can vary from mild to severe and include irritability, agitation, euphoria, and depression. Mood swings and insomnia can also be side effects. Memory loss can occur, but clears when dosage is adjusted.

Increased susceptibility to infections. As high doses of steroids suppress the immune system to reduce the symptoms of lupus, the body may not be able to defend itself against infections such as pneumonia.

Stomach discomfort. Peptic ulcers can develop, although they can be minimized by taking the drug with meals or along with medications that prevent stomach damage.

Aggravation of preexisting conditions. Corticosteroids can cause or aggravate diabetes, glaucoma, cataracts, and high blood pressure. They also often increase cholesterol and triglyceride levels in the blood.

Side effects from long-term use and high doses of steroids can be more severe. Dr. Katz advises careful monitoring for cataracts, avascular necrosis of the bone, osteoporosis, and premature arteriosclerosis.

Cataracts. Cortisone can spontaneously bind to proteins such as the collagen in the lens of the eye. This "caramelizes" the lens, which results in the clouding called cataracts.

Avascular necrosis of bone. This condition results from the death of bone due to lack of circulation to that particular area. This produces pain, an abnormal bone scan, and an atypical x-ray appearance. It occurs most often in the hip, but can also affect the shoulders, knees, and other joints. Removal of a core of bone to reduce increased pressure within the bone or total surgical joint replacement may be necessary for pain relief.

Osteoporosis. Thinning of the bones can occur because steroids reduce calcium absorption in the gastrointestinal tract. Osteoporosis

Steroids and Children

Dr. Jimmy Lawrence believes that the treatment of lupus is no different for children than for adults. "The commonly used corticosteroids," he says, "can cause stunted growth in children, which is a real concern, but in both children and adults the use of these drugs should be minimized whenever possible."

can lead to bone fractures, especially compression fractures of vertebrae, causing severe back pain. Calcium supplements and other medications may help prevent or treat this problem.

Premature arteriosclerosis. There is a relationship between steroids and a narrowing of the blood vessels by fat (cholesterol) deposits. Cholesterol levels should be checked periodically and elevated levels treated with effective new medications such as statins.

Not everyone who takes corticosteroids struggles with these side effects. In fact, some have no problems at all. Unfortunately, it is impossible to predict who will and who will not tolerate this treatment (although dosage is always an important factor), or even which side effects to expect. For these reasons, although steroids are extremely effective in the management of many lupus symptoms, treatment should always be closely monitored by your doctor and kept at the lowest possible dose.

If your doctor prescribes corticosteroids, Dr. Daniel Wallace advises taking some preventive tactics to minimize the side effects:

- Take antacids or other medications recommended by your doctor (such as Zantac or Prilosec) to counter stomach problems.

- Diuretics can be used to deal with bloating and fluid retention.

- Calcium supplements can protect bone health.

- Mild sedatives can help manage sleep problems.

- Exercise can help minimize muscle atrophy and osteoporosis.

- Avoid people with colds or other infections to reduce the risk of stressing the immune system.[11]

It's also important to know that you should never stop steroid treatment suddenly. When synthetic steroid hormones are introduced into the body, the adrenal glands may "turn off" their own production of those hormones. Stopping the drug suddenly can result in having no cortisone in your body at all, which can be life threatening. For this reason, the dosage of steroid medication should be gradually reduced over time, so the adrenal glands can slowly return to full function. To prevent a total shutdown of the adrenal glands, some physicians prescribe an alternate-day treatment plan in which the drug is taken every other day, allowing the adrenal glands to remain functioning. During the stress of surgery, higher doses of steroids will be given to you intravenously to prevent a drop in blood pressure or metabolic changes.

Immunosuppressive Drugs

Immunosuppressive drugs, which, as the name suggests, suppress the immune system, are known by a variety of names. They may be called by the rather frightening word "chemotherapy," or by the encouraging label "steroid-sparing," or by the simple term "cytotoxic." Whatever label a physician chooses to use, when lupus is severe or threatens the health of major organs such as the kidneys, it is often treated with this category of drugs, which includes Imuran (azathioprine), Immunex (methotrexate), and Cytoxan (cyclophosphamide). These drugs can be of great value in the treatment of lupus because they can help to prolong life, preserve organ function, reduce symptoms, and sometimes even put the disease into remission. They also help to reduce the need for high-dose steroids, which can increase the risk of side effects that may be worse than the disease itself. Immuno-suppressive drugs can be used either in addition to, or instead of, steroids, or they may be used to lower the amount of steroids needed (which explains the label "steroid-sparing").

In his article "Imuran, Cytoxan, and Related Drugs," Dr. Katz says that because of the way these drugs affect cell growth they are especially helpful in cases where the kidneys or other major organs are involved. "Cells in the body divide and grow at varying rates," he explains. "Examples of rapidly dividing cells include the antibody-producing cells of the immune system, blood cells, hair cells, gonadal cells, and malignant cells. Cytotoxic (*cyto* means cell, *toxic* means damage) drugs work by targeting and damaging the cells that grow at a rapid rate. In lupus, the immune system is hyperactive and produces auto-antibodies at a rapid rate of growth. Cytotoxic medicines have their greatest effect against rapidly dividing cells and, therefore, can be beneficial in the treatment of lupus by suppressing activity."[12]

Cyclophosphamide (Cytoxan) is one of the immunosuppressive drugs that are commonly used in the treatment of organ-threatening lupus. Neil Kurtzman, M.D., University Distinguished Professor in the Department of Internal Medicine at Texas Tech University Health Sciences Center in Lubbock, Texas, says that cyclophosphamide therapy is typically administered by injection. (It can be given in pill form orally, but this form can cause a severe inflammatory disease of the bladder, so it is avoided if possible.) "It is usually given along with steroids once a month for about 6 months," says Dr. Kurtzman. "There have been studies done in the last 10 years that have demonstrated that this treatment is more effective than giving just steroids alone. This is an advance in treatment because before we had cyclophosphamide therapy,

> ## The Scoop on Vaccinations
>
> Because lupus medications suppress the immune system, some people worry about receiving vaccinations. But Neil Kurtzman, M.D., feels it is not necessary to avoid them. "There is no evidence to support the idea that vaccinations can cause a flare of lupus symptoms," he says.

75 percent of patients with severe lupus nephritis could be expected to lose kidney function within 5 years, even when treated with steroids. This is no longer the case."

Cytoxan is well tolerated by most people, but because it is a potent chemotherapy drug that is used to treat a whole variety of forms of cancer, it can have serious side effects. As it suppresses the immune system, you may be more likely to develop infections. It can cause hair loss and stomach upset and exacerbate shingles (a painful, blistering skin condition caused by the herpes-zoster virus). Since it depresses bone marrow, Cytoxan can cause decreases in white blood cell, platelet, or red blood cell counts. It can also increase the risk of cancers such as leukemia and bladder cancer, and cause temporary or permanent sterility in both women and men.[13] In fact, premature ovarian failure is a significant complication that occurs in up to 60 percent of women over 30 years of age.[14] Oral Cytoxan can cause bleeding from the bladder.

> *Before we had cyclophosphamide therapy, 75 percent of patients with severe lupus nephritis could be expected to lose kidney function within 5 years, even when treated with steroids.*
>
> —NEIL KURTZMAN, M.D.

Imuran (azathioprine) is another immunosuppressive drug often used in the treatment of lupus. It is less potent and less effective than Cytoxan. But, although like Cytoxan it can decrease the blood counts and increase the risk of developing lymphoma, it has fewer side effects and is considered safer than some other immunosuppressive drugs.

Methotrexate has been quite effective in controlling joint inflammation in patients with rheumatoid arthritis. Due to its safety and effectiveness, it is now used to treat lupus.

Other cytotoxic drugs related to cyclophosphamide are chlorambucil (Leukeran) and nitrogen mustard (Mustargen). These drugs have similar immunosuppressive activity and side effects. Other promising immunosuppressives currently available include the leukemia drug 2-chlordeoxyadenosine (2-CDA), a recently approved rheumatoid arthritis drug leflunomide (Avara), mycophenolate mofetil (CellCept), and cyclosporin A (Neoral and Sandimmune), a drug also used to prevent organ transplant rejection.[15]

If you have severe lupus, immunosuppressive drugs can be a lifesaver. Your doctor will consider what is called the risk-benefit ratio to decide if the benefits of taking the drug outweigh the risks. If so, you will need close medical supervision to prevent risky side effects, monitor your blood count, and adjust the dosage as needed.

Dr. Kurtzman cautions that, even with this kind of potent therapy and careful medical supervision, the prognosis for severe lupus is variable. "It depends on the other manifestations," he says. "Patients typically have more than one organ system involved and it depends on how severe that involvement is. Every patient is different from any other. Lupus is a serious disease and even with aggressive treatment some people still get kidney failure. Although there have also been major advances in the way we understand the complicated immune system (which offers hope that we'll eventually get at the cause), because the immune system is so complicated, with multiple interactions, we still have a long way to go."

> *If you have severe lupus, immunosuppressive drugs can be a lifesaver. Your doctor will consider what is called the risk-benefit ratio to decide if the benefits of taking the drug outweigh the risks.*

The Trial-and-Error Approach to Medications

Sheri, 42, is the managing editor of an online health Web site. She has lupus and has spent years looking for just the right treatment. Her first symptoms of lupus, in 1992, were skin rashes on her legs and scalp, joint pain in her hands, knees, and feet, and mouth sores. These symptoms would come and go and would be especially difficult to manage if she went out in the sun. Five years and several doctors later, she was diagnosed with lupus, after which her doctor immediately prescribed the corticosteroid prednisone. "I really hate being on that drug because of the side effects," says Sheri. "So now my rheumatologist uses it as a stopgap measure for about six days when I'm in a flare. But initially, I used this drug a lot—once for over a year."

Of course, everyone reacts differently to each drug, but for Sheri, even at the low dose of 6 milligrams, the side effects of prednisone are difficult to live with. "The most obvious side effect for me," says Sheri, "has been weight gain and puffiness. I now weigh more than I ever have in my life. I get the double whammy of increased appetite and then bloating as well. It also makes me very hyper and I've learned that I can't make any major decisions when I'm on prednisone because I'm not emotionally able to make good choices. It's like having a really bad case of PMS. The worst side effect is that I now have osteoporosis and have broken several bones in the last few years. Also, because prednisone suppresses the immune system, I always get some kind of infection when I'm on it, but because the medication masks symptoms of infection like fever and pain, I don't know I'm sick until I go off it or until the infection is really advanced. Once I had a kidney infection that we didn't know about until I went off the prednisone and then had to be admitted to the hospital."

Despite its benefits, Sheri was not able to bear the side effects, so after 2 years her doctor switched her to the antimalarial Plaquenil. "Although I experienced no side effects from this drug, after about 3 months it was clear that I was gaining no benefit either," remembers Sheri. "So during my next flare, my doctor gave me the immunosuppressive drug methotrexate. I had to wait 6 weeks before I could expect any results, but it was well worth the wait. This drug has been amazing. I've gone into complete remission with few side effects. I feel nauseous the day and maybe the day after I take the drug (I take it once a week), and my hair started falling out (which could be from the drug or from the lupus itself), but still the results were worth it. I was on methotrexate for about 8 months and then I stopped taking it because I was feeling great and didn't want to be on such a strong drug for too long if it wasn't necessary."

Then Sheri was in a car accident that sent her into a bad flare and so she went back on the methotrexate. "My doctor feels I should stay on methotrexate," says Sheri, "until some other equally effective drug or therapy is introduced. Although some people have bad side effects with this drug, compared to the prednisone, I would take methotrexate any day. I'm on a low dose, and aside from the nausea and having to be careful about not having alcohol and not being exposed to infection, I have no problems with this at all and it has helped me tremendously. I'm also careful to stop for a week or so if I get a cold, a sore throat, or any other type of illness. Because methotrexate is an immunosuppressive drug, it suppresses my ability to fight off infection. I need to let my body do what it's supposed to do when I'm sick. And I don't go into my six-year-old daughter's classroom in the winter when everybody is coughing and sneezing. Even the people I work with have been really great about understanding when I need to work at home."

> *My doctor feels I should stay on methotrexate until some other equally effective drug or therapy is introduced. Although some people have bad side effects with this drug, compared to the prednisone, I'd take methotrexate any day.*
>
> —SHERI

Sheri also takes 150 milligrams of DHEA every day (see page 88 for information about DHEA). Her doctor didn't suggest it, but she didn't discourage it either when Sheri asked her advice. "I started taking 100 milligrams and didn't notice much difference in my health. But when I bumped it up to 150, I really felt better. And now I've noticed that when I stop taking it or when I use a cheap brand from an unknown company I feel much worse."

In addition, Sheri takes preventative action. "I now use the nasal spray miacalcin and 1,500 milligrams of calcium to counter the osteoporosis, and because I have the blood clotting problem associated with lupus, I also take an aspirin and 1,000 milligrams of vitamin E every day. I've also learned that I have to be religious about avoiding the sun. Sun exposure has made me sicker than any other kind of trigger. Even when I'm taking sun precautions, I sometimes still pay the price. Once

I went out on the golf course and had forgotten to put sunscreen on the back of my neck and that sent me into a very bad flare."

Although Sheri says she feels "wonderful," being realistic, she admits that during 25 to 30 percent of each year she feels "really miserable." She still has joint pain almost every day (especially during a cold winter) and lives with the chronic fatigue common to lupus. "I still can't go through a whole day doing whatever I want without stopping to rest, and I don't think I feel like a 42-year-old should feel. Although," says Sheri with a laugh, "I've never been 42 before, so maybe this is how I'm supposed to feel—but I don't think so!"

SUCCESS STORIES

Tiffany, 25, who, if you recall from the previous chapters, has lupus nephritis, is very much aware of the benefits, as well as the side effects, of immunosuppressive drugs. "As soon as my doctor realized that my kidneys were in bad shape, I went into the hospital to begin treatment and my doctor told me I had three options. The first and most effective was an immunosuppressive drug called Cytoxan, but the side effects were so harsh I was afraid to try it. I'm only 25 years old and I'm about to get married. He told me that this could send me into early menopause and make it impossible to have children. My fiancé and I decided that instead we'd try another regimen that was supposed to be almost as effective. I began large intravenous doses of the corticosteroid methylprednisolone for one week to try to shock the inflammation. At the same time, I began taking a milder immunosuppressive called Imuran that I'll take for the next 3 years. This has worked very well without any side effects. Since I started this treatment about 6 months ago, every test result that I've gotten back (I get tested every few weeks) has shown improvement and the last one showed that the kidney inflammation was completely gone. It's been very positive. I feel wonderful. I'm very fortunate that the problem was caught in time and I'm doing so well."

Kim, 24, who works in a public relations firm, is also doing very well after being treated for lupus nephritis—even though her treatment protocol is different from Tiffany's. When Kim was diagnosed with lupus with kidney involvement at the age of 17, her doctor immediately prescribed 60 milligrams of prednisone daily along with 150 milligrams of oral Cytoxan daily. "My doctor wanted to treat this very aggressively and put out the forest fire, so to speak," says Kim. "I didn't experience the side effects that I know these drugs can cause, but I was still worried. My doctor told me that because of the steroid, I could gain about 50 to 75 pounds. Fortunately, he also told me that if I avoid salts, sugar, and fats (which are metabolized differently because of the lupus) that probably wouldn't happen, and he was right. I created all kinds of new and improved things to eat with no added salt, fat, or sugar and I've stayed at 121 pounds the whole time (although my face did get a little puffy). I stayed on the Cytoxan for about 2 months and on the prednisone for almost a year (it took that long to wean off the steroids slowly as my doctor reduced the dosage little by little). Then I went into remission and was completely off all medications (except for blood pressure medicine that I need due to the kidney damage).

My doctor told me that because of the steroid, I could gain about 50 to 75 pounds. Fortunately, he also told me that if I avoid salts, sugar, and fats that probably wouldn't happen.

—TIFFANY

"Then about a year later I had a relapse and started the same treatment and diet again. This time I had more side effects. I had no energy; I was always tired; I was nauseous a lot; my hair started falling out; and my face was a lot more swollen. I've always handled things pretty well, but this time I was frustrated. I didn't want to go through this again, but I had no choice."

After another year on the medications, Kim again went into remission and, due to what her doctor calls some kind of miracle, she has had no signs of the disease and has taken no medication for 3 years now. "I have been very lucky," laughs Kim. "The medical treatment my doctor prescribed has worked very well for me."

In the Future

Patients with lupus are doing much better today than they were 30 years ago, but the current treatment is not like taking penicillin for syphilis and getting cured. But there are drugs under study that may eventually get us to that point. I'm working on a drug study that is designed to look at flares of lupus nephritis. (In theory, this drug may work for all manifestations of lupus, but that's not what we're specifically looking at right now.) In mice, this drug seems to *prevent* kidney damage so that looks very promising.

—*NEIL KURTZMAN, M.D.*

DHEA: UNDER INVESTIGATION

The FDA has not approved a new drug for the treatment of lupus in 40 years, but it has given priority review status to Aslera (prasterone), made by Genelabs Technologies, as it works its way through the regulatory system waiting for final approval. This designation is given to drugs that offer treatment for a disease that is severely debilitating or life threatening for which the current treatment is deemed to be inadequate. Aslera contains prasterone, which is the synthetic equivalent of the androgenic hormone dehydroepiandrosterone, or DHEA, a weak male hormone found naturally in the body. (In research papers, you may have seen Aslera referred to as GL701.)

"Lupus is one disease in which sex hormones and gender are quite important," notes Robert G. Lahita, M.D., Ph.D., professor at St. Vincent's Medical Center at New York Medical College, in his article, "Sex Hormones and Lupus Erythematosus." "Hormones may be potent regulators of cytokine levels and, consequently, disease activity." Dr. Lahita calls this function of hormones a "fundamental biologic mechanism," and although researchers may not understand precisely why these hormones affect the course of lupus, research shows that they do. Estrogens apparently contribute to disease activity, while androgens offer some protection.[16]

How DHEA Works

Before her lupus diagnosis, Darnell Samuelson had fever, joint pain, and fatigue—what felt like a constant case of the flu. She began treatment that included corticosteroids, but found that they made her jittery and caused sleeping problems. Her rheumatologist, Philip Mease, M.D., of Minor and James Medical Center in Seattle, Washington, approved her enrolling in a study using DHEA. Samuelson's lupus symptoms improved and, with the help of her doctor, she eventually was able to cease taking steroids altogether.[17]

While Samuelson's improvement was more dramatic than that of others on DHEA, well-documented studies suggest that DHEA can indeed help some people. The advantage of the drug Aslera over a placebo was consistent among the clinical trials. Flares (characterized by increased disease severity) occurred in 24 percent fewer patients who received Aslera than those who received the placebo. In addition, certain specific symptoms associated with SLE, including muscle pain, nasal and mouth ulcers and hair loss, occurred less frequently among those taking Aslera. Also, people who had been taking steroids for at least 6 months prior to entering the study showed increased bone density after taking Aslera. (As stated previously, steroids are known to decrease bone density, potentially leading to osteoporosis.)[18]

Potential Risks of DHEA

DHEA is considered safe, with no significant side effects reported in women who took as much as 200 milligrams every day for a year. Doses as small as 25 milligrams a day may decrease your levels of good (HDL) cholesterol, however, and may cause acne and growth of facial hair.

Nonprescription DHEA

Even before the FDA approves DHEA for the treatment of lupus, you can find DHEA in over-the-counter supplements in pharmacies, health food stores, and even in warehouse discount stores. Because the FDA or any other organization does not regulate such supplements, however, no guarantee exists of what you are actually getting.

"These preparations contain varying amounts of DHEA," says Dr. Ronald van Vollenhoven, M.D., Ph.D. "I am very reluctant to recommend any of these preparations for patients with lupus." Instead, until DHEA is available as a prescription drug, your doctor can write a prescription for DHEA to be compounded (mixed) by the pharmacist. You may have to call around to find a pharmacy that offers this service, or ask your doctor. And then ask about the cost up front. Some users have found that the pharmacies that offer this service do not accept their prescription medicine insurance.

TREATING THE SKIN PROBLEMS OF LUPUS

In some cases, the only organ affected by lupus is the skin (the body's largest organ!). As explained in chapter 1, this type of lupus is called discoid lupus erythematosus (DLE) or cutaneous lupus. In other cases, those who have systemic lupus with arthritis and organ involvement also have skin problems as part of the disease process. In fact, it is estimated that more than 90 percent of people with systemic lupus erythematosus will have some type of skin problem.[19] Therefore, the treatment of the skin manifestations of lupus is an important part of the lupus treatment.

The American Academy of Dermatology guidelines for the treatment of the skin manifestations of lupus include four levels:

- Topical treatment
- Systemic therapy

- Evolving therapies
- Surgical treatment[20]

This section takes a look at each of these.

Topical Treatment

The first line of therapy is topical treatment on the lupus lesions. Your doctor will probably first recommend the daily use of a sunscreen preparation that provides at least 15 UVB sun protection factor (SPF), as well as significant broad-spectrum UVA protection. (UV stands for ultraviolet.) Both UVB and UVA sunrays are known to cause and worsen the skin lesions of lupus, so this is an important first step.

The first line of treatment for the skin manifestations of lupus is topical anti-inflammatory treatment on the lesions.

The next type of topical treatment you might try is topical corticosteroid cream or ointment. These are available over the counter at pharmacies or even grocery stores, but most likely your doctor will want you to use a prescription-strength product. These are steroid preparations that reduce inflammation and can suppress activity of the immune system. Anthony Gaspari, M.D., a dermatology professor at the University of Maryland School of Medicine, adds that a topical corticosteroid medication can also be delivered to the skin lesion through a corticosteroid-impregnated tape. "This is a tape applied to the skin that has a steroid incorporated into the matrix of the tape material offering a slow release of medication," he explains. "The tape stays on for one day and is then replaced by a new tape."

If these topical treatments are not effective, your doctor may use intralesional injections of corticosteroids directly under the skin. Dr. Gaspari explains, "This is a slow release method of steroid delivery at the site of the injection that typically lasts 4 to 5 weeks and then may be repeated." Intralesional corticosteroid injections can be especially

Sun-Protected Clothing

There are new products that will help you avoid sun exposure. Two popular clothing products include:

- Rit Sun Guard is a new laundry additive that washes sun protection into clothing and helps block more than 96 percent of the sun's harmful UV rays from reaching the skin. The Skin Cancer Foundation has awarded Rit Sun Guard Laundry Treatment its seal of recommendation, as has the Good Housekeeping Institute. When added to a regular wash load, Sun Guard washes into your clothes a skin-saving SPF of 30 that provides continuous protection against damaging rays for 20 washes or more. It has no other effect upon clothing, and is safe for even the most sensitive skin. Look for Rit Sun Guard in the laundry aisle at a supermarket, drugstore, or discount store in convenient one-ounce, single-wash packages. Get more information at www .ritsunguard.com.

- Clothing that is 30+ SPF sun protected is available from a company called Solumbra. There are only a few stores around the country, but you can get a catalog or order online through their Web site at www .sunprotection.com.

useful in preventing further hair loss in otherwise unmanageable DLE lesions of the scalp.[21]

Systemic Therapy

If the skin lesions are too numerous or not responding to topical treatments, it is likely that a physician will add systemic treatment as well. The American Academy of Dermatology suggests the use of certain oral medications.

As first-line systemic therapy, this organization recommends:

- Antimalarials. Hydroxychloroquine sulfate (200 to 400 milligrams per day), chloroquine phosphate (250 to 500 milligrams per day), and quinacrine hydrochloride (100 to 200 milligrams per day).

- Dapsone, a sulfone class drug, (100 to 200 milligrams per day).

- Prednisone (0.5 to 1.5 milligrams per kilogram of body weight, per day) tapered over 6 to 8 weeks. Important note: Because of side effects, long-term use of systemic corticosteroids such as prednisone is not advisable in patients whose clinical disease is limited to the skin. Patients who do use this drug should be monitored for corticosteroid side effects (see discussion of steroids earlier in this chapter).

Second-line systemic therapies (which may be used if the other anti-inflammatory or suppressive agents are unsuccessful) include:

- Retinoids (an analog of vitamin A), especially useful in hypertrophic DLE.

- Gold (a metallic element used in the form of its salts, especially in the treatment of rheumatoid arthritis and lupus), including auranofin, gold sodium thiomalate, and aurothioglucose.

Third-line systemic therapies (which should be limited to use in patients with severe disease or disease unresponsive to other types of therapy) include:

- Corticosteroids such as prednisone (0.5 to 1.5 milligrams/kg per day).

- Cytotoxic immunosuppressive agents. Azathioprine (1 to 2 milligrams/kg per day), methotrexate (7.5 to 25 milligrams per week), or cyclophosphamide (1 to 2 milligrams/kg per day).

Sun Tips

Follow these 10 tips to avoid a skin flare:

1. Do not sunbathe.

2. Avoid unnecessary sun exposure, especially between 10:00 A.M. and 4:00 P.M. in summer or in southern climates; these are the peak hours for harmful UV radiation.

3. When outdoors, use sunscreens rated SPF 15 or higher that block both UVA and UVB rays. Apply them liberally, uniformly, and frequently.

4. Apply sunscreen at least 30 minutes before you go outside.

5. Don't forget to cover easy-to-overlook places such as the backs of your hands, tops of your feet, and your neck and throat.

6. Throw away last year's sunscreen. It may not work!

7. See your car dealer to get a tint put on your car windows. Keep the top on and the sunroof closed!

8. When exposed to sunlight, wear protective clothing such as long pants, long-sleeved shirts, broad-brimmed hats, and UV-protective sunglasses.

9. Stay away from artificial tanning devices.

10. Get covers for fluorescent bulbs to restrict UV radiation indoors.

Evolving Therapies

Evolving or experimental oral medications need further study, but are showing some promise in the treatment of skin problems associated with lupus. According to the American Academy of Dermatology, these include clofazimine, interferon alfa-2a, and thalidomide. Although Dr. Gaspari is reluctant to use interferon alfa-2 or clofazimine due to lack of scientific backing, expense, and possible side effects, he is particularly interested in the positive possibilities of thalidomide. "I would have to say that this is not a treatment in evolution anymore. In my personal opinion, thalidomide should be moved up from the category of evolving agent to a second- or third-line agent. As long as patients are compliant with specific safeguards against birth defects in pregnant women and possible nerve damage, it can be a very effective therapy."

Surgical Treatment

Surgery is a possible treatment for the scars, pigmentation changes, and hair loss resulting from healed lupus skin lesions. For example, Dr. Gaspari says that a dermatologist might use procedures such as dermabrasion or excision to reduce the size or severity of scars. These procedures can replace an irregularly shaped, raised scar with a more cosmetically acceptable, thin, linear scar.

Dr. Gaspari also notes that a surgical procedure called epidermal autografting can be successfully used to replace unsightly white (depigmented) areas of scar tissue. A study out of the Postgraduate Institute of Medical Education and Research in India reported successful "skin transplants" in three males and one female with DLE by taking healthy skin from the upper thigh and grafting it to depigmented areas of the face. The color match was good and there was no loss of pigment or recurrence of the disease during the follow-up of 6 months to 1 year. Studies such as these confirm that the scars of healed inactive DLE lesions can be successfully treated with epidermal grafting.[22]

Another approach to the treatment of lupus lesion scars is an evolving treatment using a laser treatment called erbium:yang laser. A recent study out of the department of dermatology at McGill University in Quebec sought to assess the safety and efficacy of laser resurfacing in the treatment of facial scars in DLE. This study describes a case of a 66-year-old woman with a 25-year history of relapsing DLE who developed extensive scarring on her face. After being treated with erbium:yang and followed for more than 2 years, it was found that the woman showed remarkable cosmetic improvement with no further scarring or reactivation of her disease.[23] This is another procedure with great promise for the future.

Surgery is also often successfully used to treat alopecia, localized balding. Dr. Gaspari has used scar revision procedures to help his patients with permanent hair loss due to scarring on the scalp. "The goal," he says, "is to reduce the size of the scar so that there is more healthy skin where hair can grow. I think this is a reasonable and acceptable treatment for this problem of hair loss."

Alopecia can also be treated with epidermal autografting, which is literally a scalp transplant. "The dermatologist can take a 'plug' of hair-bearing scalp, like from the back of the head," says Dr. Gaspari, "and transplant it into the scarred area so hair can once again grow there."

The skin damage caused by lupus lesions can be severe and difficult to treat. As Dr. Gaspari says, "I try to help my patients under-

---

Rheumatologist or Dermatologist?

If your skin lesions are severe, you might wonder if your rheumatologist is the right person to provide treatment. Dermatologist Anthony Gaspari, M.D., feels that rheumatologists in general do very well with the skin manifestations of autoimmune diseases. He says, "Some rheumatologists are very comfortable treating skin problems and they know the appropriate therapies like topical treatments and sunscreens. But others are less so. It's a good idea to work with a team that includes both a rheumatologist and a dermatologist if you have major concerns about skin or scalp problems."

stand that there will not be quick results no matter what methods of treatment we use. These treatments require a lot of patience and it's important to have realistic expectations."

HOPEFUL SIGNS IN LUPUS MANAGEMENT

Today's advancing and evolving medical therapies for both SLE and DLE, ranging from skin creams to injections, from oral medication to skin transplants, offer much hope for improvement and treatment options in the management of lupus. But because there is no medical treatment guaranteed to ease any of the symptoms of lupus, many people look to complementary and alternative treatments as well. The next chapter explores some of these therapies and examines how they can be used to manage lupus.

CHAPTER 4

Complementary and Alternative Therapies

$\backsim$

I F YOU HAVE lupus, you probably also have a cabinet full of prescription medications. These often lifesaving treatment regimens are the first line of defense in your battle to maintain your health. But, like Henrietta Aladjem, a founder of the Lupus Foundation of America, who traveled far and wide in her pioneering quest for treatment for her lupus, you may be willing to try just about anything that might bring relief because conventional medicine doesn't have all the answers. That's why many people with lupus turn to complementary and alternative medicine (CAM), health therapies that are not fully accepted by the conventional medical community.

Tantalizing tales of "cures" abound—you may hear of someone who avows that a certain type of juice cured her lupus, or another who says that using magnets has made all the difference. Many people with lupus have turned to acupuncture, hypnosis, or massage for relief. So, you may be wondering, what works? What doesn't? What could be dangerous?

Many different types of therapies can help in various ways. A combination of both scientific research and anecdotal evidence shows that CAM has helped some people with lupus reach the goal of relieving inflammation and pain. This chapter explores the treatment possibilities of acupuncture, herbs and supplements, massage, chiropractic, CranioSacral therapy, homeopathy, and magnet therapy. This is not an all-inclusive list; there are many other CAM possibilities out there you might want to try. The ones discussed in this chapter will give you a place to start.

BE CAUTIOUS

There are many legitimate and effective complementary and alternative therapies for the treatment of lupus. There are also many that teeter on the edge between legitimate and unproven, and await further study. And, of course, there are also many that are no more than fraudulent quackery. If you decide to give complementary and alternative medicine a try, you'll need to do a bit of investigating first. Here are a few first steps to keep in mind:

- In each type of CAM, the system of licensing practitioners varies from state to state; to find a trained and competent therapist, you should contact the national organization, if one exists, for a sound referral.

- Gather as much information as you can on the therapy you're interested in from reliable sources such as the Arthritis Foundation, the Lupus Foundation, the National Institutes of Health, or universities or hospitals. The Internet can be a great resource because many of these groups have Web sites packed with information and research (see the appendix for Web site addresses), but be careful because there are also many sites that are loaded with false information.

- Ask friends and others for specific referrals to practitioners.

- Don't expect miracles. Because no two people are identical, either physiologically or psychologically, a therapy that works wonderfully for one person may affect a second person differently. The acupuncture, for example, that apparently brings healing relief to one person with lupus may have little or no effect on another.

- Discuss CAM possibilities with your doctor. She may not agree with the potential benefits, but she absolutely must know what you're doing in order to be a committed member of your health team. (Also, never discontinue or reduce doses of prescribed medication without the guidance of your doctor.)

- The fees for these services vary from one practitioner to another and insurance coverage is never a sure thing. Some insurance companies will cover CAM, others cover it in certain circumstances, and still others will not touch it. Find out how much a therapy is going to cost you before you find yourself in debt.

PLOT YOUR PROGRESS

When you use CAM to treat the various symptoms of lupus, take it slowly. If you try multiple therapies at the same time, you'll have no way of know what is working and what is not. In the article, "Using

---

Questions to Ask a CAM Practitioner

Before you begin any CAM therapy ask the practitioner:

- Does the therapy you use help people with lupus? What evidence do you have?

- Have you treated patients with lupus? May I talk to them?

- How much will this therapy cost, and how many visits will be necessary before we know whether it's working?

- Could this therapy interfere with my conventional care?

- Are you willing to discuss your plans with my medical doctor?

Alternative Treatments," Pat Randolph, director of psychological services at Texas Tech Medical Center's pain clinic advises, "If you're thinking of trying more than one type of alternative therapy for your condition, don't try them all at once. Evaluate one first, then another, either alone or combined with the first (if your doctor agrees that the combination is safe)."[1]

A good way to do this evaluation is to plot your progress carefully. Ask the CAM therapist or doctor if there are objective ways to meas-

Sample Entries in a Symptom Diary

Keeping a daily symptom diary will help you assess your progress. Rate your symptoms on a 0-to-10 scale and note any additional information that might be relevant.

May 12

Joint pain: 8

Fatigue: 9

Muscle tenderness: 7

Skin rash: 10

Notes: Beginning new medication, twice daily, once before breakfast and once before bedtime.

June 12

Joint pain: 4

Fatigue: 9

Muscle tenderness: 5

Skin rash: 10

Notes: One month after beginning new treatment, I can feel a significant difference in my joint and muscle pain with no side effects. Unfortunately, my fatigue and skin rash remain unchanged.

ure improvement in your condition. If so, have any necessary tests or measurements taken before starting the treatment you've chosen. Also, note how bad your symptoms are, using a scale of 0 (no symptoms) to 10 (unbearable). During treatment, keep a daily symptom diary (see sidebar), again using the 0-to-10 scale, adding any specific details that seem important. After a month or two, review your symptom diary with the CAM practitioner and have any necessary tests or measurements done to assess your progress. This should give you a good idea of whether you're getting any real benefit from the treatment.

ACUPUNCTURE

Virginia Carpenter was diagnosed with lupus after her first miscarriage. She struggled through the next 15 years with many lupus-related health problems, then landed in the hospital after a major flare-up. Her doctors told her that her lupus would next move to her brain, and she had perhaps a year left to live. This was harsh news, especially considering that Virginia was a widow with two young children she didn't want to leave orphaned.

A friend encouraged Virginia to see an acupuncturist in Santa Fe, which was 65 miles from her home in Albuquerque. Although Virginia knew next to nothing about acupuncture, at that point she was willing to try anything. Unfortunately, at the time, Virginia felt so weak and fatigued that traveling 65 miles was something akin to climbing Mount Everest. She made and canceled several appointments until finally she was able to travel to Santa Fe and begin acupuncture treatments.

"It saved me," she says simply. Today, Virginia inline skates, works out at the gym, and has 20-minute Japanese acupuncture sessions once a week. And, most important, she has outlived the prediction of her death by a decade and a half. Conventional science can't confirm that acupuncture is an effective treatment for lupus, but Virginia is absolutely sure it has helped her.

"The whole idea is that you are helping to activate healing mechanisms within the body," says Robert Hayden, an acupuncturist in

Evanston, Illinois, who specializes in Japanese acupuncture (the type Virginia uses) and has treated many people with lupus. "It's not just for pain—it acts on the body's inner mechanism, to adjust itself back into a balanced state of health."

Acupuncture was little known in the United States until 1971. Following President Richard Nixon's historic visit to China, *New York Times* reporter James Reston wrote about the procedure that helped alleviate abdominal pain after Reston had surgery in Beijing. Since then, acupuncture has grown in popularity dramatically in the Western world. A 1993 FDA report estimated that Americans spent $500 million on 9 to 12 million visits to acupuncture practitioners annually.[2] In 1995, there were an estimated 10,000 nationally certified acupuncturists, according to the National Institutes of Health, and that number is expected to have doubled by now. And most interesting, currently an estimated one-third of certified acupuncturists in the United States are medical doctors.[3]

> **Resource Referral**
>
> To get more information about the possible role of acupuncture in the treatment of lupus, contact:
>
> **Lupus Acupuncture Network**
> 8808 Harwood
>   Avenue NE
> Albuquerque, NM
>   87111
> Phone: (505) 298-9550

How Acupuncture Works

According to the traditional Chinese medicine model (in which acupuncture is a primary treatment), your life energy, called *qi*, is made up of spiritual, emotional, mental, and physical aspects of life, and travels through your body via pathways called meridians or channels. Blockages at certain points along the meridians correspond to the health of specific regions of your body. The theory is that acupuncture needles unblock obstructions and reestablish the healthy flow of qi.

Practitioners of traditional Chinese medicine believe that if the flow of your qi is interrupted, the forces of yin and yang become unbalanced, and illness may result. Taoist philosophy says that yin and yang are opposite forces; when they are working in harmony, a body is healthy. If the balance is upset, disease can result.

"You can think of yin as the things in your body that keep it cool, and yang as the ones that keep it warm," says Al Stone, a licensed acupuncturist in Santa Monica and West Hollywood, California. "In traditional Chinese medicine, lupus is associated with a deficiency of yin," he explains.[4]

In acupuncture, hair-thin needles are inserted shallowly into the skin at specific points on the body (called *acupoints*). Japanese acupuncture includes moxibustion, in which therapeutic herbs (often mugwort) are burned atop the acupuncture needles. This form of acupuncture is more hands-on than standard Chinese acupuncture, in which needles may simply be inserted and left for periods of time. "In Japan, acupuncture and bodywork or massage therapy are often practiced together," Robert Hayden explains.

Some researchers theorize that the pain relief or anesthetic effect from acupuncture results from a natural response to the insertion of the needles. Some evidence indicates that your body releases endorphins (the body's natural painkillers) when acupuncture is performed, or that acupuncture somehow influences other body chemicals. Other research suggests that acupuncture alters blood circulation, increasing your blood flow to the thalamus, the part of your brain that relays pain messages. By whatever mechanism, acupuncture is a well-established method of pain management.

What to Expect

On your first visit, the acupuncturist will likely do a lengthy interview, asking details about your health and lifestyle. Be honest and specific about your health history, symptoms, any medications you take, and any other therapies you are using.

While your health particulars will determine the specifics of your treatment, treatments generally include placement of three to 15 needles, which remain in place for 15 to 40 minutes. No wonder everyone who considers using acupuncture wants to know, "Does it hurt?" The American Academy of Medical Acupuncture says that people experience medical acupuncture needling differently, but most people feel only minimal sensation as the needles are inserted; some feel nothing at all. No pain is felt once the needles are properly in place. Because acupuncture needles are very thin and solid and their points are smooth, as opposed to hollow needles with cutting edges like hypodermic needles, insertion through the skin is not painful, like injections or blood sampling are.[5] "In Japan, there's a saying that a good acupuncturist should be able to needle a sleeping cat without disturbing it," says Hayden, who studied in Japan and is certified by the National Commission for the Certification for Acupuncture and Oriental Medicine.

Safety Guidelines for Acupuncture

Acupuncture is generally safe, but as with any therapy, you should be cautious. The following guidelines are adapted from *The Arthritis Foundation's Guide to Alternative Therapies:*

- Get a diagnosis from a medical doctor before undergoing acupuncture to make sure you don't have a condition requiring prompt medical attention.

- Don't stop your medications without consulting your doctor. Acupuncture can work with, rather than instead of, conventional medicine.

- Tell the acupuncturist about all health conditions, including pregnancy. Stimulating certain acupuncture points, particularly those on or near the abdomen, can trigger uterine contractions and could induce premature labor and possibly miscarriage.

- Tell the acupuncturist about all medications you are taking. Some herbs, nonsteroidal anti-inflammatory drugs, and, of course, anticoagulants, can cause you to bleed easily even when thin acupuncture needles are inserted. You should also consult your physician before having acupuncture if you are on such medication.

- Don't take muscle relaxants, tranquilizers, or painkillers right before acupuncture because acupuncture can intensify the effects of these drugs.

- Because you have a compromised immune system, be sure the acupuncturist uses disposable needles.

- Electrical stimulation of acupuncture needles, which is sometimes used to stimulate acupoints, could cause problems for people with pacemakers (as can magnets).

- If you have diabetes, the practitioner should insert needles into your limbs only with extreme caution. Even a small skin cut in a person with diabetic neuropathy can turn into a severe infection.

- Tell the practitioner right away if you experience pain. Acupuncture shouldn't hurt after a possible initial sting with the needle's insertion.

Finding an Acupuncturist

For a list of accredited acupuncturists, contact the following organizations:

National Certification Commission for Acupuncture and Oriental Medicine
Phone: (703) 548-9004
E-mail: info@nccaom.org
Web site: www.nccaom.org

American Academy of Medical Acupuncture
This organization offers a list of medical doctors and osteopathic physicians.

Phone: (800) 521-2262
Web site: www.medicalacupuncture.org

- Do not automatically take herbs offered by traditional Chinese medicine practitioners. They can interact with prescription drugs.[6]

Finding an Acupuncturist

As acupuncture becomes increasingly popular in the United States, medical doctors are becoming familiar with the procedure and its practitioners. In fact, it is a licensed health profession in 39 states and in the District of Columbia. If you choose to try acupuncture, ask your doctor for a referral to a practitioner or contact one of the national acupuncture organizations for a referral.

When you find a practitioner you are interested in, ask if he or she is certified by the National Certification Commission for Acupuncture and Oriental Medicine (and look for this certificate in the practitioner's office—it should be displayed proudly!). In some states, you may find practitioners with a Doctor of Oriental Medicine (D.O.M.) or Oriental Medical Doctor (O.M.D.) degree. If your state requires licensing, look for a practitioner who is licensed. If your state does not, ask if the acupuncturist has qualifications from another state or what training he or she has completed.

Once you begin, track your progress. If you have no response at all after four to six sessions, this therapy may not work for you. Or you may want to try another acupuncturist because, as in any therapy, skill levels vary.

HERBAL MEDICINE

Herbal remedies are no longer considered by most Americans as some sort of voodoo medicine. They are a rapidly growing, mainstream business; U.S. users spent an estimated $3.65 billion for herbal remedies in 1998, which was a 100 percent increase since 1994.[7] It is likely that you or your friends may have a few bottles of herbal supplements in your cabinet right now; advertisers tell us to buy *Ginkgo biloba* (ginkgo) for brain power, St. John's wort for depression, and echinacea for colds and flu. And yes, some herbs are recommended for the treatment of lupus symptoms—but with caution.

Four Herbs for Lupus

Research has suggested that the herbs frankincense (*Boswellia serrata*), ginger (*Zingiber officinale*), turmeric (*Curcumin longa*), and ashwagandha (*Withania somniferum*) can provide pain relief. For thousands of years these four herbs have been used in Ayurvedic medicine (the traditional medicine of India) to treat arthritis and other pain ailments. Optimal benefits apparently result when the herbs are used together.

There is some scientific backing behind the use of these herbs to reduce joint pain. Research reported at the American College of Rheumatology annual scientific meeting in 1998 looked at a remedy incorporating these four plant extracts. In a randomized double-blind trial of 90 people with osteoarthritis, those patients who took the combination experienced significant and sustained pain relief: 50 percent improved, compared to 20 percent of those who took a placebo.[8]

> *The group taking the herb formulation had improvement in pain, stiffness, and function, and few side effects.*

A 2000 study conducted at the Center for Rheumatic Diseases in Pune, India, found similar results. In a double-blind placebo-controlled trial that lasted for 16 weeks, 182 people with active rheumatoid arthritis took either the herb mix or a look-alike placebo. The group taking the herb formulation had fewer swollen joints, statistically significant improvement in pain, stiffness, and function, and few side effects. Tests that measure disease activity also showed improvement.[9]

The herb mix used in the above studies is sold commercially as Artrex. Let's take a closer look at these four herbs.

Ashwagandha *(Withania somniferum).* The roots of this Asian plant (which is related to the potato) have long been used to treat various medical conditions. A review of the literature by researchers out of the Los Angeles College of Chiropractic in 2000 found strong support for the healing properties of this herb. Of particular interest to those with lupus are the research findings indicating that ashwagandha possesses anti-inflammatory, antistress, antioxidant, immunomodulatory, and rejuvenating properties. Toxicity studies concluded that the herb appears to be safe.[10]

Ginger *(Zingiber officinale)*. This herb is widely accepted as a treatment for nausea, but a few studies indicate its role in reducing swollen joints and pain in people with arthritis. Research suggests that ginger root inhibits the production of prostaglandins and leukotrienes, which are involved in pain and inflammation. In an uncontrolled 1992 Danish study, 56 people who had either rheumatoid arthritis (RA), osteoarthritis (OA), or muscular discomfort took powdered ginger. All of those with musculoskeletal pain and 75 percent of those with OA or RA reported varying degrees of pain relief and no side effects, even among those who took the ginger for more than 2 years.[11]

Frankincense *(Boswellia serrata)*. From the gum of the boswellia tree, this herb has been shown to inhibit the production of leukotrienes, which cause inflammation.

Turmeric *(Curcumin longa)*. A few studies have credited this herb with causing some reduction in swollen joints and pain in people with arthritis. With no significant side effects, it apparently inhibits prostaglandin production and stimulates the creation of cortisol, which can help relieve inflammation.[12]

Other Possibly Helpful Herbs

There is some evidence that St. John's wort, ginkgo, and feverfew may also help reduce the symptoms associated with lupus.

In *The Lupus Book*, *Dr.* Daniel Wallace notes that "controlled studies suggest that St. John's wort has mild serotonin-boosting properties that might aid fatigue and depression, while ginkgo may improve cognitive dysfunction."[13]

The herb feverfew has long been used to relieve the pain of migraine headaches and may work inside cells to block inflammatory action. But use it with care. In his article, "Is Feverfew a Pharmacologic Agent?," George Wong, M.D., notes, "There is wide variation in the quantities of active compound in individual plants, plant parts, and fresh and dried preparations. As is the case for other proprietary

Beware of Scams

Whenever a product promises complete relief or a "cure," be extra cautious. Some scientific evidence suggests that increasing your intake of certain vitamins and minerals can help relieve lupus symptoms—and you'd better believe that plenty of marketing folks read those findings with dollar bills in their eyes.

You will find many concoctions or special diets advertised to help your lupus, most with hefty price tags attached, and some with vigorous accolades from anonymous sources. "I have SLE lupus," declares an unidentified woman on one company's Internet site. "I was bedridden for 3 years and for the next 3 after that I was just dragging myself around. That all changed in October when very good friends gave me 'Product X.' "

Perhaps this is a very real woman who did get wonderful benefits from her "Product X." However, it's best to copy down all ingredients of products and other company information and ask your doctor's advice before you jump on the bandwagon. Remember that the Food and Drug Administration does not regulate supplements, so you have no guarantee as to what a certain pill or potion contains, or even if it is safe. You might also check out companies with the Better Business Bureau in your area.

herbal medications, some commercial feverfew products have been found to contain little or no active phytocompounds. Therefore, only standardized extracts should be used." Wong also warns, "There are no studies documenting feverfew's long-term safety or efficacy."[14] If you choose to give this herb a try, it is generally agreed that it should not be used with other pain medications. In addition, because of the lack of long-term safety data, the Canadian Health Protection Branch (HPB) recommends that feverfew not be used for more than 4 months without medical supervision. The HPB also warns that abrupt discontinuation of this herb can result in muscle and joint stiffness and nervous system problems such as rebound pain, anxiety, and poor sleep patterns.[15]

Use Herbs with Care

Joanne Forshaw of Lancashire, England, was diagnosed with lupus in 1996. Since that time she has become what some might call a lupus activist. She coordinates a lupus information forum; produces an informational Web site, The Lupus Site, at www.uklupus.co.uk; and is on the committee of the Lupus UK Lancashire & Cheshire Regional Group. She often writes about alternative and complementary care for lupus symptoms, but always with a word of caution. Here is her best advice:

Natural isn't necessarily safer. Natural substances can contain powerful, potentially toxic chemicals. Just because a product is labeled "natural" or is from a plant source, it is not guaranteed to be safe.

Herbal supplements are virtually unregulated. Unlike prescription and over-the-counter drugs, which must pass rigorous, multiphase testing to receive approval, herbal supplements are exempt from this process and are not regulated. Manufacturers are not required to divulge the full list of ingredients in these products. Therefore, people are not fully aware of how much or even what substances they are consuming. Anyone with lupus should know, for example, that some Chinese herbal preparations contain potent steroids and some contain sulfa derivatives and other substances that trigger allergic reactions in most people with lupus.

Beware drug interactions. Some herbs cannot be taken along with certain medications. Mixing some herb-based products with medication (either prescription or over-the-counter) may cause a host of unexpected interactions and side effects that can be very dangerous.

Avoid alfalfa. Alfalfa sprouts contain an amino acid known as L-canavanine, which has been known to increase inflammation in patients with autoimmune disease. All members of the legume family contain L-canavanine, but it is highly concentrated in alfalfa. Many people with lupus have no trouble eating alfalfa sprouts, but have a flare response if they ingest a supplement containing alfalfa in which L-canavanine is highly concentrated; in fact, many food products and some "natural" vitamin remedies contain L-canavanine, so be sure to read labels and avoid this substance.

> *Natural substances can contain powerful, potentially toxic chemicals. Just because a product is labeled "natural" or is from a plant source, it is not guaranteed to be safe.*

Avoid echinacea. Echinacea is known to boost the immune system and therefore boosts the autoantibodies that are your enemies. People with lupus should avoid this herb. Echinacea appears in many herbal remedy preparations, so always read labels and avoid any products that claim to boost the immune system.

Talk to your doctor. Remember always to consult your physician before using any nonprescription remedies, and never stop taking prescription drugs without talking to your physician first.

Although some people with lupus have found relief from herbal medicines, almost all herbal practitioners and medical doctors agree that herbs alone cannot treat the symptoms of lupus. "Yes, these herbs work," says D. Edwards Smith, M.D., a rheumatologist and Ayurvedic

---

Drug Interactions You Should Know About

The Arthritis Foundation cautions you to remember that herbs and other supplements can be powerful medicine: "herbal" and "natural" do not mean "gentle" or "harmless." Before you consider any supplement or herb, review its possible interactions or side effects. For example, keep in mind that ginkgo, ginseng, and fish oil can all increase the effects of blood-thinning drugs; ginger can increase the side effects of nonsteroidal anti-inflammatories; and zinc can interfere with glucocorticoids and other immunosuppressive drugs.[16]

---

practitioner who is now dean of the Maharishi College of Vedic Medicine in Albuquerque, New Mexico, "but herbs are just one part of therapy."[17]

NUTRITIONAL SUPPLEMENTS

You may find some symptom relief from certain nutritional supplements that contain healthy oils or fats, particularly fish oils and flaxseed oil.

Fish Oils

EPA (eicosapentaenoic acid) and DHA (docosahexaenoic acid) are the most important omega-3 essential fatty acids (EFAs) in certain fish oils. Studies have found that fish oils with these EFAs have a number of medical benefits. They appear to lower triglyceride levels, raise HDL ("good") cholesterol, "thin" the blood, reduce levels of homocysteine (an amino acid), slow down atherosclerosis, perhaps treat hypertension, and effectively treat the early stages of rheumatoid arthritis.[18]

Researchers have also conducted studies specifically on the use of fish oils in the treatment of lupus symptoms. One small double-blind placebo-controlled crossover study, conducted over 34 weeks, compared a placebo against daily doses (20 grams) of EPA from fish oil. Of the 27 individuals who completed the trial, 14 showed improvement when taking EPA, while the 13 receiving the placebo were rated as worse or having no change.[19] Researchers conducting another double-blind study at Victoria Hospital in London, Ontario, followed people with lupus kidney disease for more than 2 years, and found that those taking fish oil showed some signs of improvement. At lower doses (6 grams), the fish oil reduced inflammation; at higher doses (18 grams), it altered the mechanisms responsible for both inflammation and clogged arteries.[20]

Flaxseed Oil

Flaxseed oil contains omega-6 and omega-3 essential fatty acids (but a different type of omega-3 from the EPA and DHA in fish oil). It also contains plant lignans and alpha-linolenic acid, which have various functions in your body and can help ease symptoms of Raynaud's phenomenon and other lupus symptoms. In a study at the University of Western Ontario in London, Ontario, nine people with lupus kidney disease received 15 grams of flaxseed oil a day for 4 weeks, then 30 grams for 4 weeks, and then 45 grams for another 4 weeks. The researchers concluded that 30 grams of flaxseed daily was a safe dose that improved kidney function and reduced inflammation. Researchers theorize that flaxseed oil may act against a platelet activator that causes some lupus symptoms.21

> **Try the Real Thing**
> Fish oil and flaxseed supplements are a quick way to increase your EFA intake, but don't overlook the natural sources in your diet. The best choices are fatty fish such as salmon, albacore tuna, and mackerel. Flaxseed can be ground into meal and used in baking or as a cereal topping.

Gamma-Linoleic Acid

Gamma-linoleic acid (GLA), is an omega-6 essential fatty acid found in borage oil, black currant oil, and evening primrose oil. As with other fatty acids, our body uses GLA to make various substances that influence inflammation and pain. GLA may help you make prostaglandins and leukotrienes that block inflammation and protect your heart, although the effect specifically for lupus is untested. A few small studies suggest GLA may help with Raynaud's phenomenon.[22]

MASSAGE

Massage, like acupuncture, has been used to treat various ailments for thousands of years. Chinese medical texts dating back 4,000 years mention massage, and it has played a part in Western medicine since the time of Hippocrates. In the United States, massage has moved in and out of favor in the medical community, but it is now recognized as a valid method of medical treatment. Primary care physicians are increasingly referring patients to massage therapists for complementary care. The American Massage Therapy Association (AMTA) reports that according to a survey by the State University of New York at Syracuse more than half of primary care physicians stated that they would encourage patients to pursue massage therapy as a treatment. Renslow Sherer, M.D., director of Cook County Hospital HIV Primary Care Center in Chicago, told the American Massage Therapy Association, "Massage therapy has clearly been shown to me to be very beneficial, particularly in areas where conventional medicine has not been as successful."[23]

> **Check the Label**
>
> To help ensure that you are getting a safe supplement, the FDA suggests that you look for the initials "USP" on the label. This indicates that the manufacturer has followed United States Pharmacopoeia standards.

A "Last Resort" Turns Into a Lifetime Vocation

In the early 1970s, Mary-Jo Myers was very sick. At first she was treated with antibiotics for flu symptoms—achy muscles, fatigue, and fever. But nothing helped; in fact, one of the antibiotics caused ulcerative colitis and sent Mary-Jo to the hospital for a month! The symptoms grew worse and worse until Mary-Jo became critically ill, left her job at a pharmaceutical company, went on disability, and was eventually bed and wheelchair bound. Due to connective tissue breakdown, Mary-Jo could not lift her feet (she slid them along the floor) or raise her arms to bring her hands any higher than her mouth. Finally in 1974, Mary-Jo went to a hematologist who analyzed blood tests and diagnosed systemic lupus erythematosus. The doctor told Mary-Jo that this was a fatal disease (which it often was at that time). What terrible news for a woman in her early thirties with two children aged five and six.

"In the course of my early treatment, I was on over 60 different medications," remembers Mary-Jo. "But nothing was working. I had a strong faith in my Creator and I kept praying that something would happen that would let me raise my two precious children, but it seemed I was asking for a miracle."

The answer to her prayers came in the form of a chiropractor that Mary-Jo had gone to over the years for back pain. She had stopped going when she became what she thought was terminally ill. Curious about her "disappearance," this chiropractor went to her house, listened to her story, and then announced, "I'm going to help you." Mary-Jo had her doubts and was not anxious to let him waste his time trying to save her. But then he said, "Do you think you're dying?" Mary-Jo answered, "I know I am." "Well, then," he asked, "what do you have to lose?" So Mary-Joe reluctantly began chiropractic treatments and, also at his recommendation, called on a friend who was a massage therapist to work with her also. This decision turned her health and her life around.

"I began a deep muscle massage treatment call Pfrimmer Deep Muscle Therapy. This was founded in Canada by a woman named Therese Pfrimmer, who sat in her own wheelchair and cured herself of paralysis using this method. My friend, the massage therapist, went to Canada to study this technique and came back to help me. After about only four sessions, my range of motion was restored and I was out of the wheelchair; I could feel my whole body slowly responding and getting better. Still, it took me about a year to accept that I might really live to see my children grow up. Eventually, I gave up all medications and have never gone back to them. The way my body has responded to this massage has just been amazing.

"That's when I decided that I wanted to use my business background to help my friend establish a business giving this massage therapy to others in need. We started with one table in the basement of my home. Within 18 months, we could not accommodate all the people who wanted to schedule appointments. We realized that we needed to train other therapists so that people in all different parts of the country could enjoy the benefits that I had. So we established the first school of massage in the tri-state area around Pennsylvania. It took 3 years of fighting with the local authorities. But finally in 1982, we opened our doors. Now we have a beautiful building housing the Pennsylvania School of Muscle Therapy in Oaks, Pennsylvania, with over 30 employees. We teach the Pfrimmer deep muscle massage, as well as basic and medical massage. We also now have a degree program in affiliation with a local college and offer an associate degree in muscle therapy and integrative health care."

Obviously, Mary-Jo has outlived her doctor's fatal predictions almost 30 years ago. "I still have lupus," she says; "I still have my deep muscle massage at least once every 2 weeks and reflexology twice a week, and still there are days when I don't feel very well and have to take it easy. But I'm now 66 years old and have three wonderful grandchildren that I never expected to see, and I have this business that is helping other people, so I am a happy and blessed woman."

Types of Massage

The National Institutes of Health (NIH) defines massage as "the scientific manipulation of the soft tissues of the body to normalize those tissues. It consists of a group of manual techniques that include applying fixed or movable pressure, holding, and causing movement of or to the body, using primarily the hands but sometimes other areas such as forearms, elbows, or feet. These techniques affect the musculoskeletal, circulatory-lymphatic, nervous, and other systems of the body. The basic philosophy of massage therapy encompasses the concept of *vis medicatrix naturae*—that is, aiding the ability of the body to heal itself."[24]

This is a general definition, covering the basics of massage. If you explore massage as an alternative therapy, you'll find that there are many different types. The NIH divides the 80 different methods of massage therapy into three major groupings:

> **Point-and-Click Referrals**
>
> You can find an international listing of alternative health professionals on the Web site www.holistichealthcare.com.

Traditional European methods are based on traditional Western concepts of anatomy and physiology, using five basic categories of soft-tissue manipulation: effleurage (gliding strokes), petrissage (kneading), friction (rubbing), tapotement (percussion), and vibration. Swedish massage is the main example of this type.

Contemporary Western methods are based on modern Western concepts of human functioning, using a wide variety of manipulative techniques. These may include broad applications for personal growth, emotional release, and balance of the mind, body, and spirit in addition to traditional applications. These methods go beyond the original framework of Swedish massage and include: neuromuscular, sports, and deep-muscle massage; and myofascial release, myotherapy, Bindegewebsmassage, Esalen, and manual lymph drainage.

Structural, functional, and movement integration methods organize and integrate the body in relationship to gravity through manipulating the soft tissues or through correcting inappropriate patterns of movement. These methods bring about a more balanced nervous system through creating new integrated possibilities of movement. Examples are Rolfing, Hellerwork, Aston patterning, Trager, Feldenkrais, and the Alexander technique.[25]

How Massage Can Help You

Whatever the name or type, it is clear that massage is much more than a relaxing luxury. Research has shown that massage has a variety of medical benefits. The American Massage Therapy Association notes that massage "reduces heart rate, lowers blood pressure, increases blood circulation and lymph flow, relaxes muscles, improves range of motion, and increases endorphins. Therapeutic massage enhances medical treatment and helps people feel less anxious and stressed, relaxed yet more alert."[26]

In the past 50 years, more than 100 clinical trials have been published about massage and its health benefits. Although no studies yet have focused specifically on lupus, massage is known to relieve many of the associated symptoms of lupus, including chronic pain, chronic inflammation, muscle spasm, anxiety, depression, and insomnia.[27]

Finding a Massage Therapist

You will find massage therapists in private practice, at the local gym, spas, hair salons, or even at the mall. But finding the one who is best for you and your special lupus needs will take a bit more investigating because the benefit you receive from massage therapy depends on the skill and training of the therapist.

Do not use the Yellow Pages to find a therapist. Inconsistencies in national accreditation and licensing make it difficult to obtain a guarantee that everyone listed in the phone book is really a trained therapist. It's also risky because, unfortunately, some shady escort services advertise under the heading of "massage." The best method of finding a good therapist is through a medical or word-of-mouth referral. You can also find a trained and experienced therapist by checking for professional backing, training, and licensing, such as the following:

- The American Massage Therapy Association has more than 40,000 members in more than 20 countries. This organization has existed since 1943 and requires its members to follow a code of ethics and standards. Members must be graduates of accredited training programs and have a minimum number of classroom hours.

- Certification by the National Certification Board for Therapeutic Massage & Bodywork is an indication that a massage therapist has attained the highest professional credential in the field. Look for a therapist who has this certification.

- The District of Columbia and 25 states have state regulatory boards that require special registration and licensing, so check out licensed massage therapists through your state's health department.

Resource Referral

You can find a trained and licensed massage therapist by contacting:

American Massage Therapy Association
820 Davis Street, Suite 100
Evanston, IL 60201
Phone: (847) 864-0123
Fax: (847) 864-1178
Web site: www .amtamassage.org

Potential Risks of Massage

You should always check with your doctor before seeking a massage. According to the American Massage Therapy Association, therapeutic massage can be inappropriate with certain health conditions, including:

- Inflammation of the veins (phlebitis)
- Infectious diseases
- Some forms of cancer
- Some skin conditions
- Some cardiac problems[28]

CHIROPRACTIC

The word *chiropractic* means "treatment by the hands or manipulation." It is a system of healing developed by David Daniel Palmer in 1895. Palmer believed that displacements of the spine caused pressure on nerves, which created pain or symptoms in other parts of the body.

Chiropractic treatment and patient management includes a variety of procedures used in accordance with the treating doctor's education, experience, and best clinical judgment. These include (but are not limited to) chiropractic adjustments, manipulation, mobilization, physiotherapeutic modalities and procedures, exercise rehabilitation, nutritional counseling, ergonomics advice, and supportive appliances. Chiropractors use x rays and orthopedic and neurological tests in the diagnostic process.

A chiropractic treatment, which is drug-free and nonsurgical, often focuses on adjustment and manipulation. Adjustments involve dynamic thrusts (rapid, precise, and painless force) to a specific vertebra in order to remove any interference with nerves. Manipulations are more general reorderings of bones to realign joints and increase a person's range of motion.[29]

Studies have found that therapeutic manipulation has a role in the management of various chronic conditions including fibromyalgia (which shares the symptoms of pain and fatigue with lupus). One study included 15 adult members of a regional fibromyalgia association who received chiropractic treatments including ischemic compression and spinal manipulation. The researchers found that 30 treatments reduced the intensity of the participants' pain, sleep disturbance, and fatigue. They also found that the improvement in all three measures was maintained after 1 month without treatment.[30]

If you decide to give chiropractic medicine a try, it is important to choose an experienced chiropractic doctor through a medical or personal recommendation because chiropractic treatment involves highly specific adjustment of the spinal tissues. Always be certain that your chiropractor is state licensed and reputable. Never allow a "paraprofessional" or other unlicensed per-

Resource Referral

You can get a referral to a trained chiropractor in your area by contacting:

American Chiropractic Association
1701 Clarendon Boulevard
Arlington, VA 22209
Phone: (800) 986-4636
Web site: www .amerchiro.org.

son to attempt a spinal manipulation; this could worsen your problem rather than help it.

CRANIOSACRAL THERAPY

Osteopathic physician John E. Upledger developed CranioSacral Therapy (CST) following extensive scientific studies from 1975 to 1983 at Michigan State University where he served as a clinical researcher and professor of biomechanics. CST involves gentle pressure and manipulation of the craniosacral system, composed of the skull, spine, and the fluid that flows around the brain and spinal cord. Misalignments in this craniosacral system can cause pressure on the bones, which in turn can affect the rate of flow of this fluid. When the flow rate is "off," health problems can develop. CST works on making delicate adjustments to the spine or bones of the head to correct the flow rate.

Celina Klee of the Upledger Institute, in Palm Beach Gardens, Florida says, "CST is a gentle, hands-on method of evaluating and enhancing the functioning of a physiological body system called the craniosacral system. . . . It enhances the body's natural healing processes and has been effective for a wide range of medical problems associated with pain and dysfunction including lupus. There is no way to tell if an individual patient will benefit, but advanced CST therapists have noticed good results with many of their SLE patients. Since CST is very gentle and noninvasive, it can be a good thing to try."

> **Resource Referral**
> You can find a CranioSacral therapist by contacting:
>
> **Upledger Institute**
> 11211 Prosperity Farms Road, D-325
> Palm Beach Gardens, FL 33410
> Phone: (561) 622-4334, ext. 1335

HOMEOPATHY

Homeopathy is a system of health care and treatment developed in the 1800s by Dr. Samuel Hahnemann. The philosophy of homeopathy is based on Dr. Hahnemann's research with natural medicines in which he found that "like cures like." A substance causing certain symptoms in a healthy person can cure a sick person with the same symptoms. This theory is based on the belief that the body enlists its own energies to heal itself and defend against illness. If a remedy that causes symptoms similar to those of the illness is administered, the body steps up its fight against it, thereby promoting cure.

Homeopathic remedies are derived from plants such as aconite or dandelion; from minerals such as iron phosphate, arsenic oxide, or sodium chloride; from animals, as in the venom of certain snakes or the ink of the cuttlefish; or even from chemical drugs such as penicillin or streptomycin. The remedies are prepared through multiple careful dilutions of the substance until little of the original remains.

Resource Referral

To find a practitioner licensed in homeopathy, contact:

National Center for Homeopathy
801 North Fairfax
   Street, Suite 306
Alexandria, VA 22314
Phone: (877) 624-0613
   or (703) 548-7790
Fax: (703) 548-7792
Web site: www
   .homeopathic.org

The National Center for Homeopathy (NCH) tells us that, although most homeopathic medicines are available without a prescription, they are drug products made by homeopathic pharmacies and that (unlike herbs) their manufacture and sale are closely regulated by the FDA. Each individual state regulates the practice of homeopathy. Usually it can be employed legally by those whose degree entitles them to practice medicine in that state. This includes the M.D. (medical doctor), D.O. (doctor of osteopathy), N.D. (doctor of naturopathy), D.D.S. (dentist), and D.V.M. (veterinarian) credentials. Homeopathic practitioners can also include chiropractors, nurse practitioners, physician assistants, acupuncturists, and certified nurse midwives.[31]

Homeopathy is an individualized therapy. A practitioner takes a detailed history of your health, lifestyle, preferences, and symptoms to determine your "constitutional type," which indicates the homeopathic remedy that is appropriate for you.

The beauty of homeopathy is that there are no side effects and it can be used with conventional treatments. Jennifer Jacobs, M.D., on the faculty at the University of Washington in Washington State, has been using homeopathy for 23 years in her medical family practice. She told *Arthritis Today* that many of her patients take conventional medicine along with homeopathic medicine, and some find that they can gradually reduce their conventional medication—but this should be done *only* under a doctor's care, she cautions. Dr. Jacobs also notes, "Acute ailments such as the flu or a stomach upset may clear up with one dose in a few hours or days. But chronic conditions such as arthritis may take several months of treatment." Homeopathy preparations used for arthritis pain (which in many cases is related to the joint pain of lupus) include *Rhus toxicodendron* (from poison ivy), *Bryonia* (from wild hops), *Apis* (from bee venom), and *Ledlum* (from marsh tea).[32]

Be Patient

Although there are no harmful side effects associated with homeopathic remedies, practitioners say symptoms sometimes worsen briefly before they begin to get better. This is what is known as a "healing crisis."

If you decide to try homeopathic remedies, heed this advice provided by the Arthritis Foundation:

- Don't try to treat yourself if you have a systemic rheumatic disease such as rheumatoid arthritis or lupus. And don't expect homeopathy alone to be enough. Consult your regular medical doctor as well.

- Don't give up your prescription medications without your doctor's okay. It can be dangerous to stop some drugs abruptly.

- Look for a homeopath with years of experience, certification from a national homeopathic organization and, preferably, medical training.

- Use only products labeled with the words "produced in accord with the U.S. Pharmacopoeia Convention" to be sure you are getting a pure homeopathic product, not one mixed with drugs or other substances.

- Read the labels if you have alcohol concerns: Some remedies are diluted with alcohol.

- Take only one remedy at a time, and keep detailed notes about what you take and any effects you feel. This will help you determine if it appears to help your symptoms or track any adverse effects.

- Don't continue a therapy that isn't working: Homeopaths say remedies show effects for minor ailments in a few days. For a chronic disease such as arthritis, it may take up to two months. If you don't improve after that period, it's probably not the right remedy, or homeopathy may not be the right treatment.

- Remember, more is not better: The whole philosophy of homeopathy is small doses. Take the remedies as directed, in tiny amounts.

- Side effects are rare, as homeopathic remedies have little (if any) active ingredients. If you develop new symptoms, however, stop taking the remedy right away and consult your homeopath and doctor.[33]

MAGNET THERAPY

The term *magnet therapy* usually refers to the use of static magnets placed directly on the body, usually over areas of pain. Static magnets (also known as permanent magnets) are either attached to the body by tape or are held against the body in specially designed products such as belts, wraps, or mattress pads.

Although magnet therapy has recently been receiving a lot of attention, it certainly is not new. Reliable documentation tells us that Chinese doctors believed in the therapeutic value of magnets at least 2,000 years ago, and probably earlier than that. The Chinese used magnets to treat many ailments including fevers, arthritis, wounds, and pain from injuries.[34] Today, magnet therapy is becoming increasingly popular as an inexpensive pain-reliever without side effects.

During the 1970s, magnet therapy became popular among athletes from many countries for treating sports-related injuries. By the late 1990s, it was common to see a golfer wearing a magnetic wrist wrap or hear testimonials from tennis players about the value of magnetic mattress pads. But it was not until 1997 that scientific studies of magnets were reported in the United States. The results of these studies have suggested that there may indeed be therapeutic benefits from magnets.

In one particular study at the Baylor College of Medicine and the Institute for Rehabilitation and Research in Texas, Drs. Carlos Vallbona and Carlton F. Hazlewood evaluated magnet therapy in adults diagnosed with post-polio syndrome who were experiencing arthritic pain in the joints or had identifiable points of pain in their muscles. The participants were 39 women and 11 men. Because the joint and muscle pain of post-polio syndrome is similar to the type of pain some people experience with lupus, the results of this study may be of interest to you.

> *The majority of patients in the study who received treatment with a magnet reported a significant decrease in pain, and most of the patients who were given a placebo, or inactive magnet, reported very little or no improvement.*

All participants were asked to press on the trigger point where they felt the severest pain and rank that pain on a scale of 1 to 10, with 10 being the worst. The patients were then randomly given an active or inactive magnet to strap against their trigger point for one 45-minute session. The low-intensity magnets, less than a half-inch thick and slightly stronger than refrigerator magnets, were available in four formats to accommodate different areas of the body: a credit card–size rectangle, a 6-inch strip almost 2 inches wide, a disc the size of a silver dollar, and a disc the size of a CD. After the magnets were removed, participants rated the intensity of their pain again.

The 29 participants who received an active magnet had an average pain score of 9.6 before the treatment, and 4.4 after wearing the magnet.

The placebo group had an average pain score of 9.5 before treatment, and 8.4 afterwards. None reported negative side effects. "The majority of patients in the study who received treatment with a magnet reported a significant decrease in pain, and most of the patients who were given a placebo, or inactive magnet, reported very little or no improvement," Dr. Vallbona reports.[35]

These kinds of results speak for themselves, but the question remains: How do magnets work to reduce pain? "We do not have a clear explanation for the significant and quick pain relief observed by the patients in our study," says Dr. Vallbona. "It's possible that the magnetic energy affects the pain receptors in the joints or muscles or lowers the sensation of pain in the brain." Offering another possibility, Stefanie Oppenheim, Ph.D., a representative for Nikken, a research and development company that has investigated the medical use of magnets for 25 years, says, "My understanding is that the energy helps your body physiology function more optimally on the cellular level." Some other theories suggest that cell membranes benefit from magnetic stimuli, that magnets stimulate the release of endorphins, or that magnets balance your body's electromagnetic field.[36]

Whatever the mechanism of magnet therapy, it does seem to help some people manage chronic pain better. Although the long-term effects have not been evaluated, there are no immediate negative side effects of this alternative therapy, so it's something you might want to try if you live with pain. Beware of the magnet products sold without any medical guidance, however. "These products, like the bracelets and necklaces sold through magazines," says Dr. Oppenheim, "make medical claims without an explanation of their technology, their true strength, the possible side effects, or a proper way to use them, and this can be misleading. The buyer must beware."

Resource Referral

For more information about magnet therapy or to receive a referral to a magnet therapist, you can contact Dr. Stefanie Oppenheim through her Web site at www.5pillars.com /stefanieoppenheim.

A PERSONAL EXPERIMENT

Your quest for the optimal therapies to relieve the pain, skin rashes, fatigue, or organ damage of lupus is, in a sense, a personal experiment to find a therapy and a practitioner best for you. Remember that no treatment yet available for lupus offers a cure, only possible relief. Be sure you are choosing a treatment that fulfills the venerable doctors' credo for treatment: "Do no harm." The next chapter will increase your complementary treatment options to include both nutrition and exercise.

CHAPTER 5

Nutrition and Exercise

❧

AFTER YOUR DOCTOR has prescribed whatever medications he or she feels will help relieve your lupus symptoms, and after you've investigated alternative and complementary therapies, giving some a try and deciding against others, your lupus treatment continues to require your active involvement. Now you can begin to make up your own diet and exercise plan, personally tailored to make you feel better. No one can make you include diet and exercise in your daily treatment, but if you do, you'll be giving your body what it needs to defend itself against an autoimmune attack.

EATING FOR LUPUS RELIEF

There is no official diet recommended for people with lupus. Dietitians, physicians, researchers, and medical writers, however, consistently agree that you will benefit from a well-balanced, nutritious diet. Most of us know that we should be eating healthful foods, and understand that dining on fast-food burgers, fries, and shakes several times a week isn't accomplishing this. But we're bombarded by advertisements for fast-food fixes and processed foods, and enticed by jumbo-size bags and boxes of food at warehouse stores. In addition, we lead hectic, busy lives. The result is that few of us eat as well as we should.

Regardless of the obstacles, the advice to eat a well-balanced, nutritious diet still stands. For the record, eating well means the following:

- First and foremost, limit your serving sizes. For most of us, a serving of meat should be the size of a deck of cards, not a 16-ounce, T-bone steak. In general, Americans consume too many calories. Just cut back on the amount of food on your plate at every meal and see the difference in your health and your waist.

- Choose lean protein sources such as lean meat, poultry, fish, tofu, and lowfat yogurt.

- Choose whole-grain products and fiber-rich cereals instead of white bread, sweet rolls, or cereal whose first ingredient is sugar.

- Eat at least five servings of fruits and vegetables a day (the more colorful and less cooked the better).

- Limit treats such as candy, cake, cookies, and soft drinks.

- Limit fat in the diet. One tablespoon of butter, margarine, vegetable oil, or mayonnaise delivers about 100 calories and 9 to 10 grams of fat.

- Drink eight glasses of water a day.

Foods to Focus On

In addition to an all-around healthful diet, people with lupus can benefit from avoiding certain compounds in the diet that might aggravate lupus symptoms and by including more of certain substances that can help to ease symptoms. Amy Christine Brown, Ph.D., an assistant professor of nutrition at the University of Hawaii at Manoa in Honolulu, reviewed medical literature on lupus and nutrition dating from 1950 to March 2000.[1] After studying all the available material on lupus and diet during this period, she concluded, "The type of diet that might help laboratory animals with lupus may or may not benefit humans. If it did, then patients with lupus erythematosus might benefit from a balanced vegetarian diet (perhaps some fish allowed) that is portion controlled to avoid excess calories, and contains rich sources of vitamin E, vitamin A (beta-carotene), selenium, and calcium (if taking corticosteroids)."

Let's take a closer look at the nutrients that the scientific literature says may help ease lupus symptoms:

In addition to an all-around healthful diet, people with lupus can benefit from avoiding certain compounds in the diet that might aggravate lupus symptoms and by including more of certain substances that can help to ease symptoms.

Vitamin E. This vitamin is a powerful antioxidant. Although still controversial, vitamin E in high dosages (over 300 IU) appears to help alleviate rashes in some people with lupus, while in others it has no affect. You should inform your doctor if you are taking excess vitamin E because it thins the blood and is actually prescribed by some physicians for this purpose in heart patients. Food sources of vitamin E include polyunsaturated vegetable oils, seeds, nuts (sunflower seeds), and whole grains.

Beta-carotene. Because beta-carotene is an antioxidant with many healthful qualities and abounds in foods that are nutrient- and fiber-dense, it's a good idea to include these foods in your diet. This substance occurs in dark green, orange, and yellow vegetables, and is converted to vitamin A in our bodies. Good sources include carrots, carrot juice, sweet potatoes, pumpkin, spinach, romaine lettuce, broccoli, apricots, mango, cantaloupe, papaya, and green peppers.

Selenium. Our bodies use the mineral selenium to produce an enzyme that acts as an antioxidant, working with vitamin E to control dangerous free radicals. (Free radicals are highly reactive molecular fragments that bond with virtually any biological, carbon-based substance they come into contact with, weakening cells and impairing cell function.) Meat, seafood, dairy foods, and nuts contain selenium, and it is found in whole grains and vegetables (wheat germ, bran, brown rice, barley, red Swiss chard, turnips, and garlic) that have been grown in soil rich in selenium. Although one study found that South Dakota and Wyoming have selenium-rich soil, there's no easy way to know what type of soil your foods were grown in, so you may want to consider a supplement. It's a good idea to stay close to the Daily Reference Intake (DRI) for selenium, which is 55 micrograms for adults.

Foods to Avoid

Dr. Brown's literature search also revealed that diets with excess calories, excess protein, high fat (especially saturated and omega-6 polyunsaturated fatty acids), and zinc have been found to aggravate lupus in laboratory animals prone to lupus. The following provide some good reasons to reduce these factors in your diet:

Avoid excess calories and fat. "If you're a mouse with lupus," says Dr. Brown, "it is known that cutting back on calories will expand your lifetime due to the fact that kidney problems don't show up as soon. Fewer circulating immune complexes, proinflammatory cytokines, and kidney lesions occur in calorie-restricted laboratory animals. These results may or may not apply in humans."

Avoid excess protein. "Go vegetarian," advises Dr. Brown. "That seems to be the gist of the research done on mice and lupus. Simply put, low-protein diets improve survival rates in autoimmune mice. There is a delayed development of autoimmunity in lupus-prone mice if they are put on lower-protein diets. Protein in the diet is primarily found in meats, dairy, and eggs. It's important to keep to your recommended levels, which is determined by multiplying the weight you would like to be by 0.33 grams. For example, a 135-pound "desired" weight multiplied by 0.33 grams equals 41 grams of protein a day. To see how easy it is to overdo the protein, keep in mind that meat averages 7 grams per ounce; milk about 8 grams per cup; and eggs about 7 grams for each egg. Grains and vegetables provide protein, too. In general, grains deliver about 3 grams per cup or one slice of bread, and vegetables provide about 2 grams per $1/2$ cup cooked or 1 cup raw.

That gives you a general guide to regulate your protein intake and not overdue it like most Americans, who average 100 grams per day."

Avoid a high-fat diet. After reviewing the research literature on fat and lupus, Dr. Brown found, "Mice on diets with high overall fat had more severe autoimmune disease and decreased life spans. The type of fat also makes a difference. Stay away from omega-6 fatty acid food sources and steer toward omega-3 fatty acid sources (canola oil, fish, and fish oil or omega-3 fatty acid supplements). Fatty acids, depending on their type, determine if the body goes into overdrive with inflammation or reduces inflammation."

Avoid zinc. Zinc boosts the immune system and this can trigger a lupus flare-up. Dr. Brown suggests that it is a good idea to stay away from zinc supplements unless prescribed by your doctor. "In fact," she cautions, "anything that boosts the immune system, like getting sick or taking echinacea, should be avoided."

Nutrients to Support the Kidneys and Heart

Lupus, unfortunately, sometimes affects body organs, such as your kidneys and heart. If this happens, you may need to take special dietary precautions to help yourself stay healthy.

Kidney Disease

When your body metabolizes the protein you eat, chemicals such as urea nitrogen, uric acid, and potassium are produced. Your kidneys normally filter out these potentially toxic substances, but when kidneys begin to fail, they simply cannot do the job completely. Think of a clogged or torn coffee filter—it cannot keep all the coffee grounds out of the pot. The same is true of a less-than-healthy kidney. Your doctor may recommend that you restrict three substances in your diet that are tough on the kidneys:

- Protein (in meat, dairy, and eggs)
- Salt

- Potassium (found in certain fruits such as bananas, oranges, and grapefruit)

If possible, get the help of a registered dietitian by asking for a referral through your doctor.[2]

Cardiovascular Disease

Another problem related to the heart that might be a problem for people with lupus is high blood pressure associated with lupus kidney disease (normally the kidneys keep blood pressure regulated). High blood pressure is dangerous and should never be ignored because it increases your risk of having a heart attack or stroke.

If you have high blood pressure, your doctor may prescribe medication and ask you to limit your salt (sodium) intake.[3] Your doctor may also advise you to lose excess weight so the heart doesn't have to pump as hard to move that weight around. High blood pressure often drops when people who are overweight or obese lose some pounds.

A Personal Journey

Karen Kaufman, M.S., C.C.N., is a nutritionist in the Boston area who was diagnosed 11 years ago at the age of 38 with "autoimmune disease of unknown origin." After dealing with joint pain, fatigue, Sjögren's syndrome, and Raynaud's phenomenon for another 3 years, she was finally diagnosed with lupus without organ involvement. The treatment plan from her rheumatologist was typical: Start with aspirin and take it until your ears ring (a sign of overdosage); then move to NSAIDs. (The doctor also recommended the antimalarial Plaquenil, but Karen wasn't willing to take any drug that required eye exams every few months.)

"The worst part during this time was the loss of control over things I had always taken for granted," remembers Karen. "My health, my vitality, and my ability to function were all being taken away from me. I had to quit my job in sales because the fatigue was just so overwhelming. This is very hard to explain to people. I would wake up in the morning and realize that I felt like a normal person, but then after walking to the bathroom, my joints would be on fire—my ankles, my knees, my elbows, my wrists, and all my fingers hurt so badly—and I would be exhausted. No one knows what this feels like unless you've been through it. Even my mother wondered if maybe I was just depressed. I also had what I consider very bad cognitive dysfunction along with atypical migraines. I graduated college Phi Beta Kappa and I'm used to being mentally quick. Suddenly I couldn't think clearly and couldn't find the words I wanted to say. I'm glad my heart and kidneys are not affected by lupus, but I know my brain is. This is extremely difficult for me to deal with."

> *No one knows what this feels like unless you've been through it. Even my mother wondered if maybe I was just depressed.*
>
> —KAREN KAUFMAN, M.S., C.C.N.

Karen also had to adjust to the change in her physical capabilities. "Before getting lupus, I was very active physically. I could do 50 minutes of intense step aerobics with no problem. Suddenly, I couldn't walk around the block." After about 6 months of this, Karen decided she had had enough. "I decided that I was going to do everything I could to take back control of my health and my life. But I have to admit that when I said that I really had no idea that I could turn my health around to the extent that I have. The recovery for me has been more than I ever imagined."

Karen went back to undergraduate school to take some premed courses and then on to graduate school to get a master's degree in nutrition. "I was hoping to give myself the credentials I would need to make a living at a job I could do on my own terms (and do after sleeping in late in the morning when I needed to!)." During this time, Karen also began her quest to become physically fit again. "I started with just 5 minutes of aerobic exercise. It felt like I was walking on glass the pain was so bad. But I just knew that if I kept at it, I would not remain as sick as the doctors said I would always be." For the next few years, Karen took one college course at a time and went home to exercise, study, and then sleep. That's all she could do, but it was more than her doctors thought she could do.

Before getting lupus, Karen had been a vegetarian. Her studies in nutrition helped her adapt this diet to one that she feels has made all the difference in the state of her health. "There is no doctor in the world who can confirm that my diet has kept my lupus in a mild state, but every doctor I see says that he wishes other patients would approach this illness the same way. I'm not saying I'm cured. I just had a major flare with a migraine a few months ago that put me in bed, but I have to say that I function much better than the other people with lupus I've met through my work with the Lupus Foundation."

So how does Karen do it? "My diet now is primarily vegetarian and I eat only whole-grain products (no white flour or white sugar)," she says. "This is not a prison sentence; I do cheat sometimes, but this is always my goal. I also eat some fish, particularly salmon, sardines, and some tuna for the omega-3 oils that can block the inflammation process. But I definitely eliminate foods like chicken, turkey, and red meats that contain the saturated and trans-fatty acid fats, and also processed foods that contain partially hydrogenated vegetable oils. These all promote inflammation. I'd rather get my fats from the nut group and from olive oil because they contain monounsaturated fats, which are not involved in the inflammation process. I do drink skim milk, but only an organic brand because I figure that bovine growth hormones and estrogen that are found in nonorganic dairy and meat products can't be good for a disease that is mysteriously linked to hormones. Also, I can't stress enough the importance of using whole-wheat and grain products over white flour products. The vitamins, minerals, and fiber that are taken out of white flour products are just too important to do without and

> *I try to be kind to my kidneys, knowing they're vulnerable in lupus, by avoiding food substances that make them work too hard.*
>
> —KAREN KAUFMAN, M.S., C.C.N.

most are not put back in even when the label says 'fortified with essential vitamins and minerals.'

"I try to be kind to my kidneys, knowing they're vulnerable in lupus, by avoiding food substances that make them work too hard. Excess protein (from red meats, chicken, and cheese) taxes the kidneys and ultimately can speed up kidney failure. I also limit salt intake; salt retains fluid in the body and this taxes the kidneys. For people who are taking steroids, salt restriction is especially important. These medications can cause diabetes and hypertension, which are aggravated by the way salt retains fluid. For people with lupus, this is just bad. If you give up salt, you'll lose your salt appetite quickly. After four days of no salt, you'll be shocked how salty a potato chip tastes! There's salt in lots of products you have to look out for. If, for example, I eat Chinese food with soy sauce, I know I'll wake up in the morning with swollen joints; the salt in soy sauce retains that much fluid."

Karen supports her diet with some daily supplements. "I take 4 grams of ground flax per day because there is scientific data to support its ability to eliminate lupus nephritis and so I consider it preventative. I also take DHEA (100 milligrams daily) to help maintain normal levels; I think this works particularly well for my degree of lupus which is not quite mild, but not life threatening either. I also take antioxidants and I take a good multivitamin. I also take an iron supplement because I have anemia, but you have to be careful here because some people with lupus need to restrict their iron intake; this is a case in which your doctor should look at your red cell count and decide what's best for you. I also take fish oil supplements."

> *I am completely convinced that the combination of exercise, diet, and relaxation exercises are key to my continued good health.*
>
> —KAREN KAUFMAN, M.S., C.C.N.

All of these dietary changes have been extremely helpful to Karen. "I don't understand why more doctors don't mention diet to their lupus patients," she says. "We know diet affects inflammation, fluid retention, hypertension, and so on, so why not talk about it? I am completely convinced that the combination of exercise, diet, and relaxation exercises are key to my continued good health. Now I work about 40 to 60 hours a week as a nutrition consultant (on my own schedule that I can adapt to my physical needs). I am also very active volunteering for the Lupus Foundation in Massachusetts as their patient services coordinator. I just think everyone should know that you do have some control over how this disease affects your life."

How Diet Can Combat Drug Side Effects

The drugs used to treat the symptoms of lupus, as chapter 3 explained, can have serious side effects. Of course, your doctor will monitor your condition closely, and advise you on nutrient needs, but if you are taking corticosteroids, keep these basics in mind as you look for a diet that will help you deal with the possible side effects of osteoporosis, diabetes, and high cholesterol.

Osteoporosis

As discussed previously, osteoporosis is a potential problem for anyone who takes large dosages of corticosteroids over a long period of time. Researchers at the University of California School of Medicine in Los Angeles found that high doses of corticosteroids for more than 3 months reduced bone mass, regardless of a person's age, race, or gender. They recommended a treatment program of nutrient supplementation and exercise as soon as possible. "Because bone loss is most severe during the first 6 to 12 months of treatment, prophylaxis to preserve bone—with calcium, vitamin D, a bisphosphonate, and exercise—should begin as soon as the clinical situation permits rather than after the disease has been brought under control," the researchers concluded.[4]

The good news is that taking supplemental calcium and vitamin D does help. One study of 103 people taking corticosteroids, for instance, found that taking 1,000 milligrams of calcium plus 0.6 micrograms of calcitriol per day prevented steroid-induced bone loss in the lumbar spine.[5]

You can fight bone loss and breakage by including more foods with calcium and vitamin D in your diet, and increasing exercise to help strengthen your bones. Your doctor will probably advise 1,000 to 1,500 milligrams of calcium a day, along with 100 to 500 milligrams of vitamin D.[6]

Milk has about 300 milligrams of calcium per cup, while a cup of yogurt, 8 ounces of calcium-fortified orange juice, and half a cup of tofu with calcium have 250 milligrams each. Other good sources, at about 180 milligrams each, are a 3-ounce serving of canned sardines with the bones, half a cup of cooked collard greens, and 1 ounce of cheese. Other sources, not quite as calcium-rich, include cottage cheese, turnips, navy beans, and broccoli.

> *You can fight bone loss and breakage by including more foods with calcium and vitamin D in your diet, and increasing exercise to help strengthen your bones.*

Food sources of vitamin D include coldwater fish, butter, cream, egg yolk, liver, and fortified milk and cereal. Cod liver oil is packed with vitamin D—more than 1,300 IU per tablespoon. Salmon and mackerel boast about 350 IU per $3\frac{1}{2}$-ounce serving, and that amount of sardines has 270 IU. A cup of fortified whole milk has almost 100 IU. You can look on the side of your cereal box to find how much vitamin D a serving contains. You also can manufacture your own vitamin D from about 15 minutes of daily exposure to sunlight, but this can be dangerous if sun exposure puts you at risk for a lupus flare.

If you are taking steroids, you may want to consider a supplement of vitamin D, as steroids can interfere with uptake of this vitamin. "For these reasons, individuals on chronic steroid therapy should consult with their physician or registered dietitian about the need to increase vitamin D intake through diet or dietary supplements," advises the National Institutes of Health.[7]

Diabetes

Like other forms of diabetes, steroid-induced diabetes inhibits the body's production of insulin, making it difficult to keep a normal blood sugar level. High levels of sugar in the blood have potentially serious long-term results that can damage your nerves, eyes, kidneys, or more. In diabetes, it is crucial to regulate your intake of sugar and carbohydrate-rich foods to keep from overloading your circuits, so to speak. Exercise and loss of excess body weight also enhance your ability to use the insulin you make. You should contact a diabetes education program to learn how best to manage your diabetes. It can be an intricate balancing act with food, exercise, and medication, which is often too daunting—and far too important—to face on your own. Your doctor may give you a referral or you can contact the American Diabetes Association.

> **Resource Referral**
>
> To find more information about diet and lupus-related diabetes, contact:
>
> **American Diabetes Association**
> 1701 North Beauregard Street
> Alexandria, VA 22311
> Phone: (800) 342-2383
> Web site: www .diabetes.org

High Cholesterol

If you're taking steroids, it's possible that your cholesterol levels will need to be monitored. One study showed that increasing the dosage of prednisone by 10 milligrams daily caused blood cholesterol to rise 7.5 milligrams per deciliter. In this case, your doctor will recommend a lowfat diet.[8] (See "Tips to Limit Your Fat Intake" for helpful ideas.)

Eating Well with a Raging Appetite

The steroids that are often prescribed for lupus can make you exceptionally hungry. That uncontrollable hunger is real—you're not imagining it. What happens is that cortisone suppresses two glands that produce hormones in your body, the hypothalamus and the pituitary. This plays games with your appetite signal, so you feel hungry when you normally would not, and don't feel full when you should.

Tips to Limit Your Fat Intake

- Switch to nonfat milk, yogurt, and cottage cheese.

- Substitute applesauce for oil or butter in baking.

- Choose baked foods over fried.

- Munch on a bagel in the mornings rather than a muffin or doughnut.

- Have jam on your toast or bagel instead of butter or cream cheese.

- Pack sliced carrot sticks and an apple in your lunch every day.

- Have baked sliced potatoes and sweet potatoes instead of french fries.

- Slather your baked potato with salsa or cooked onions instead of butter or sour cream.

- Have tasty lentil, split pea, or bean soup for dinner instead of meat.

- Order your vegetables without butter.

- Order pasta with red sauce rather than a cream sauce.

- For dessert, try a scoop of sherbet or sorbet topped with sliced fruit.

"I try to concentrate on decreasing fat calories," says Margrey, who has lupus and who has struggled with steroid-fueled appetite. "Avoid salt and increase water intake. Keeping a written log of daily exercise programs plus what foods you eat every day works to focus your mind on exactly what you are eating and your activity level."

Here are a few other tips that can help you keep down your daily calorie count:

Plan a healthful diet. You need to get organized because your normal appetite signals no longer work properly. You will probably need the help of a registered dietitian to plan a diet that takes into account your special needs.

Plan ahead. Stock up your house with the foods that help you fight lupus and excess calories. You may find that you save money and time as well as calories when you have healthful, low-calorie foods within easy grabbing distance when you are starving for a quick bite.

Control portions. The cheapest and best tools to help you control food intake are a set of measuring cups and measuring spoons. A small scale can come in handy, too (look in any kitchen or office supply store). That bowl of breakfast cereal may actually be three servings instead of the one you thought you were eating. That handful of raisins may be more fattening than a slice of chocolate cake. And that hunk of roast beef may be enough protein for three people your size!

> *Y*ou will probably need the help of a registered dietitian to plan a diet that takes into account your special needs.

Don't skip meals. Even if you are one of those people who "can't eat breakfast," make yourself have something before you head out the door—even a glass of milk will help—or leave with a banana or a bagel in your hand. Eating three small meals and three healthful snacks will keep your body functioning most efficiently and help you avoid gorging or snacking on things that drive up the calorie count.

Avoid concentrated sweets. Sweet rolls or a gooey doughnut for breakfast can leave you ravenous an hour or so later because when you eat something sweet, your blood sugar rises quickly, but then plummets. Instead, have some oatmeal (preferably not the presweetened microwavable variety, also loaded with sugar), whole-wheat toast, or a small bagel with peanut butter.

Leave temptation behind. Clean house and office. Get rid of the box of candy in the back of your drawer and the freezer full of ice cream. Instead, fill your refrigerator shelves with chopped raw vegetables. And try popcorn (not the butter-drenched variety) when you feel the need to munch.

Food Allergies and Sensitivities

Some medical and consumer literature has proposed the possibility that lupus is caused or worsened by certain food allergies or sensitivities. These theories, however, have not yet proven true. A few proposed links you may hear about include the following.

Celiac Disease

Some researchers have claimed that lupus is exacerbated or caused by an intolerance to the gluten in wheat, rye, and barley, a genetic condition known as celiac disease. Celiac disease and lupus do share two specific antigens. In a study of 103 lupus patients at Brooke Army Medical Center in Fort Sam Houston, Texas, however, researchers concluded that no correlation existed between celiac disease and lupus.[9]

Lactose Intolerance

You may hear faint rumors of a connection between lupus and lactose intolerance, an inability to digest milk well. Robert Lahita, M.D., points out that mice with lupus have become ill when taking in milk proteins, although no evidence has been found of this in people.[10]

Aspartame

The artificial sweetener aspartame has been linked to lupus in articles that have shown up on various Web sites. These articles sound convincing; they cite doctors and use terms such as formic acid and metabolic acidosis. One article says that people who drink three to four cans daily of Diet Pepsi or Diet Coke are prone to developing lupus.

"When we get people off the aspartame, those with systemic lupus usually become asymptomatic," the article declares.[11]

This appears to be an urban legend, a modern-day myth, however, with little to no truth or scientific evidence involved. The Lupus Foundation of America consulted on this issue with Evelyn Hess, M.D., who is a leading researcher in the field of lupus, specializing in environmental influences, and then released this statement: "According to Dr. Hess, there is, as of now, no specific proof of an association with aspartame as a cause or worsening of SLE."[12]

This example shows clearly why you can't believe everything you read about lupus, especially if the information is not from an established research institute or a professional in the field.

EXERCISE: NOT AN OPTIONAL ACTIVITY

What is the last thing anyone who is tired and achy would want to do? Right—exercise. It feels like your body is crying for rest. You've convinced yourself that moving those painful joints will do more harm than good. Sitting in front of the TV seems like the perfect remedy for what ails you. But, unless you're in the middle of a flare, your body needs exercise whether it feels like it or not.

Watch out for the Effects of Alcohol

Alcohol can make arthritic symptoms worse. If you are taking nonsteroidal anti-inflammatories, alcohol can irritate your stomach. For that matter, drinking alcohol can contribute to high cholesterol, and more than two drinks a day can interfere with absorbing the calcium and vitamin D you need to protect your bones—already at risk if you have been taking corticosteroids.[13]

The Good News About Exercise

You probably know all the basic reasons why exercise is good for you. It helps keep your heart and lungs healthy and it strengthens muscles. But you may not know that exercise can have even more significant benefits for you because you have lupus. Exercise can keep your joints flexible, ease the pain, and prevent further stiffness. It strengthens your muscles so they can better protect and support your joints. It helps avoid bone loss or thinning. It builds stamina to fight fatigue. It helps keep your weight under control. And very important for people with any chronic illness, it makes you feel good and can even relieve depression. As April Jackson, M.D., a Chicago internist, says, "With any type of autoimmune disease, the patients have to exercise to maintain control; it is not an option."[14]

Getting Started

Getting started can be difficult—just the thought of walking around the block may tire you. Part of the problem is that inactivity saps your muscles of strength and conditioning. So even when your lupus isn't active, you may still feel fatigue, notes Peter H. Schur, M.D., in *The Challenges of Lupus*.[15] To get past a state of inactivity, the National Institute of Arthritis and Musculoskeletal and Skin Diseases offers excellent advice on beginning an exercise program:

- Discuss exercise plans with your doctor.
- Start with supervision from a physical therapist or qualified athletic trainer.
- Apply heat to sore joints before beginning exercise.

> **Easy Does It**
>
> Most trainers and experts recommend increasing your exercise levels no more than 10 percent per week. This is great advice. First, you need to determine what is a safe amount to start with. A walk around the block? If that seems too much, walk around your house instead. The important thing is to get started, and to do a little every day.

- Stretch and warm up with range of motion exercises.

- Start strengthening exercises slowly with small weights, even with a 1- or 2-pound weight.

- Progress slowly.

- Use cold packs after exercising.

- Add aerobic exercise.

- Consider recreational exercise. Fewer injuries to arthritic joints occur during recreational exercise if you first do range of motion, strengthening, and aerobic exercise to get yourself in the best possible condition.

- Ease off if joints become painful, inflamed, or red, and discuss this with your doctor to find the cause and eliminate it.

- Choose the exercise program you enjoy most and make it a habit.[16]

Try Hydrotherapy

Hydrotherapy (water therapy) can decrease pain and stiffness. Exercising in a large pool may be easier because water takes some weight off painful joints. Community centers, YMCAs, and YWCAs have water exercise classes developed for people with joint pain. Some people also find relief from the heat and movement provided by a whirlpool.

Exercising to Reduce Symptoms

Margrey Thompson, 46, has lupus, but that hasn't stopped her from earning a degree in physical therapy and founding her own physical rehabilitation company called TheraCare Rehabilitation Companies, based in Murfreesboro, Tennessee. Naturally, exercise has been a large part of her health regimen.

"I started feeling tremendous fatigue around age 19," remembers Margrey, "and I had a really tough time at college." But fighting through her fatigue, Margrey graduated with a degree in physical therapy and got a job as a therapist. That's when she first started having joint pain in her knees and hands. "I found I couldn't kneel on the mat tables for even 15 seconds without terrible pain," she says, "and then 6 months after I got married at age 23, I was diagnosed with lupus. Although I do have Sjögren's syndrome and Raynaud's phenomenon along with my lupus, fortunately I have never had organ involvement. I think I've stayed relatively healthy because my disease is so well managed. I have learned how to communicate with my doctors to help them help me. Last year I had to change my eyeglass prescription three times. I was sure my eye problems were related to my medication, so my doctor decreased the dosage of my prednisone from 20 milligrams to 3 milligrams and I was soon able to return to my original eyeglass prescription. My eyes are fine now. It's these kinds of small things that I am very careful on a daily basis to stay on top of. When I notice even a subtle change in my health, I put all the facts on the table for my doctor so we both always know what's going on."

Margrey also credits her health to her exercise program. "I'm learning to put myself first sometimes and take the time I need to stretch and strengthen my muscles every day. I had a flare about 1 year ago and for the past 6 months I've been stretching and using a massage therapist to work on these tender muscles. (Sometimes, I have to take a nap after a massage because it can wear me out!) I've also started walking with a group of women from the neighborhood and we've just started biking, too. (I'm hoping to get them into yoga next!) In about 6 weeks I'll start strength training, but I can't do it all at once. I've learned that I wear myself out if I do too many types of exercise at one time. We each have to acknowledge what our body is telling us and how fast or how slowly we can reach our goals. Four months ago I couldn't make my hands reach past my kneecaps; now I can lay the palms of my hands flat on the floor. I stretch when I first wake up. I stretch while I'm watching TV. I stretch every day when and wherever I can."

Margrey breaks a complete exercise program into four parts:

> I've learned that I wear myself out if I do too many types of exercise. We each have to acknowledge what our body tells us and how fast or how slowly we can reach our goals.
>
> —MARGREY THOMPSON

1. Range of motion

2. Stretching

3. Aerobic exercise

4. Strength training

She cautions, however, that you shouldn't try to do all the exercises at once. Start with range of motion and slowly work your way through stretching, aerobic, and finally, strength training.

Range of Motion Exercises

Range of motion exercises help maintain normal joint movement, relieve stiffness, and maintain or increase flexibility. "It is appropriate to put joints gently through their full range of motion once a day, with periods of rest during acute systemic flares or local joint flares," advises the National Institute of Arthritis and Musculoskeletal and Skin Diseases.[17] Talk to your doctor about how much you need to rest during flares.

Every joint in your body should be put through its range of motion. That includes neck, shoulders, elbows, wrists, fingers, waist, hips, knees, ankles, and toes. Bend them and move them all slowly through their range. Margrey recommends these three simple range of motion exercises to get you started:

Neck exercise. To move the muscles in the back and the sides of the neck, tuck your chin down to your chest while keeping your shoulders down and relaxed. Gently turn your chin up to your right shoulder, then back across your chest to your left shoulder. Be sure to keep your chin down on your chest throughout the exercise. Exhale as you rotate. Repeat 5 to 10 times in each direction.

Shoulder exercise. To put your shoulders through a range of motion exercise, put both arms straight up in the air with palms facing each other and elbows only slightly bent. Lower your arms, with palms facing down, until your arms extend out to the sides from your shoulders, each forming a 90-degree angle with your body. Repeat 5 to 10 times.

Hip exercise. Lie on your back with your knees bent and your feet flat on the floor. Keep the small of your back pressed toward the floor and keep your neck straight. Place the ankle of one leg on top of the opposite thigh (just above your knee). Inhale. Bring both legs toward your chest as you clasp your hands under the thigh of the leg that was resting on the floor. Exhale as you stretch. Hold the stretch for 5 to 30 seconds, breathing evenly while you hold. Repeat on the opposite side.

Stretching Exercises

To maintain mobility, daily stretching that exercises your trunk, neck, arms, and legs is essential," says Margrey. "Stretches must be performed in a slow, steady manner in order not to increase inflammation." Margrey recommends you begin with these simple stretches, concentrating on holding each stretch for 15 to 30 seconds (unless otherwise noted). Repeat 2 to 3 times for each body part.

> *To maintain mobility, daily stretching that exercises your trunk, neck, arms, and legs is essential.*
>
> —MARGREY THOMPSON

Low back, buttock, and thigh stretch. Lie on a firm surface on your back with your knees straight. Bend one knee up toward your chest. Hold onto your knee with both hands and gently pull the bent leg up toward your head as far as possible. Keep your lower back straight and keep your head on the floor. Relax and straighten the leg and repeat with the other leg.

Hamstring stretch. To stretch the large muscle in the back of the thigh, sit with your legs straight out in front of you and with your knees slightly bent. Stretch your arms forward and grasp your calves. Keep your back as straight as possible. Feel the stretch in the back of your thighs.

Upper chest muscle stretch. Stand up straight and face the corner of the wall. Plant both feet approximately 1 to 2 feet from the wall. Keep your stomach in, knees slightly bent, and head straight. Look straight ahead. Bend your elbows and raise your arms as close to shoulder height as you comfortably can. Place your palms on the wall (in position as if you were going to do a push-up). Slowly lean your body toward the corner. Be careful not to flex at your hips; you should press your hips slightly forward. Exhale as you lean into the wall. Hold the stretch, breathing evenly as you do and then inhale as you return to your original position.

Aerobic Exercise

When you are able, you can increase the level of exercise by increasing repetitions, adding more stretches, or by adding aerobic exercise. Aerobic exercise can improve cardiovascular fitness, help control weight, and improve overall function. Also, studies suggest that aerobic exercise can reduce inflammation in some joints. A study of people with an autoimmune disease, such as rheumatoid arthritis, at the University of Toronto in Ontario, found that exercise brought about changes in circulating immune function (including a decrease of CD4+ count [cells found in inflamed joints]) that might help regulate inflammation.[18]

> *Aerobic exercise does not have to be extremely strenuous exercise. Many people decide that exercise isn't for them and dump the whole idea because they try too much too fast and end up in pain.*
>
> —MARGREY THOMPSON

"But," cautions Margrey, "it is extremely important not to overwork yourself or you will increase the inflammatory state in your body. Start slowly with aerobic exercise, probably just a 10-minute walk a day for a week or two. Increase the time gradually until after about a month you can walk 20 to 30 minutes per session, with at least three sessions per week. But remember, when you're in severe pain, severely fatigued, or have swelling in your joints, discontinue or alter your exercise regimen."

You might also need to redefine what you mean by aerobic exercise. "Aerobic exercise does not have to be extremely strenuous exercise," says Margrey. "Many people decide that exercise isn't for them and they dump the whole idea because they try too much too fast and end up in pain. Always stretch first to loosen up your muscles and joints and then gradually build an aerobic program that you can enjoy. Walking, biking, and swimming are best for anyone with an inflammatory disease, but I recommend that everyone, especially people with lupus, avoid jogging because it's tough on the joints."

When you begin an aerobic program, think small and be proud of small gains. You can't compare yourself to anyone else, or even to your own self before lupus. You have unique health needs now; work with this fact, don't fight it.

Strength Training Exercises

Slowly add some simple strength training exercises to your program to help keep or increase muscle strength, which in turn can help support and protect your joints. "You will need to increase your muscle strength, especially in the lower extremities, shoulder girdle, and abdominal muscles," says Margrey. The National Institute of Arthritis and Musculoskeletal and Skin Diseases recommends that you do strength training daily unless you are in severe pain or have swelling in your joints.

Researchers have become increasingly interested in the benefits of weight lifting, especially for women. A 1994 study published in the *Journal of the American Medical Association (JAMA)* found that women as old as 70 could avoid the typical loss of bone—and even increase their bone mass a bit—by lifting weights twice a week for a year.[19]

Don't despair if you're not up to weight lifting, however. Strength training does not necessarily mean using free weights or machines at all. Margrey suggests you begin with these basic strengthening exercises:

> *Researchers have become increasingly interested in the benefits of weight lifting, especially for women.*

Abdominal bridge. This exercise strengthens the muscles in the buttocks, thighs, abdomen, and back. Lie on your back with your knees bent and your feet flat on the floor. Keep your stomach tight, your neck straight, and the small of your back pressed toward the floor to maintain proper alignment. Keep your arms at your sides, palms down. Inhale. Keeping your stomach tight, perform a bridging movement by pinching your buttocks together as you lift them off the floor. Exhale as you lift your buttocks. Hold the position for 5 to 10 seconds, breathing evenly. Return slowly to the starting position.

Abdominal crunch. This exercise strengthens the abdomen and the front of the neck. Lie on your back with your knees bent and your feet flat on the floor. Keep your stomach tight, your neck straight, and the small of your back pressed toward the floor to maintain proper alignment. Place your hands beside your ears with your elbows angled out. Inhale.With your stomach tight and chin tucked, slowly lift just your head and shoulders until the upper part of your shoulder blades lifts off the floor. Exhale as you lift. Hold the position for 5 to 10 seconds, breathing evenly. Return slowly to the starting position.

Easy push-up. This exercise will strengthen the muscles in the back, abdomen, neck, and arms. Lie on your stomach with your forehead resting on the floor. (Put a rolled towel under your forehead.) Place a large pillow under your stomach. Keep your hands flat on the floor at shoulder level. Inhale. Perform a push-up from the "on-knees" position, straightening your elbows as you push up. Be sure not to lock your elbows straight and try to keep your stomach tight and neck straight, so that you maintain good alignment. Exhale as you lift your body. Hold the position for 5 to 10 seconds, breathing evenly. Return slowly to the starting position.

Know When to Take it Easy

Pacing yourself is important for any exercise program, but for someone with lupus, it is crucial. "Exercise can be helpful or harmful, depending on your approach," points out Robert H. Phillips, Ph.D., author of *Coping with Lupus.* "If you throw yourself into an exercise program, you can damage untoned muscles and wear yourself out. As much as it may be contrary to your nature, you must ease into exercise and recognize when fatigue tells you it's time to back off."[20] Dr. Robert Lahita agrees: "Exercising during a flare-up is dangerous and unwise."[21] And Margrey sums it up quite simply when she says, "Just walking and maintaining your body erect against gravity during a flare is an all-out exercise program in itself."

Remember that exercise is meant to be curative and health-giving: Listen to your body and, if it's demanding rest, graciously give it what it needs. Most experts agree that if exercise causes pain that lasts for more than an hour, it is too much. People with arthritis should work with their physical therapist or doctor to adjust their exercise program when they notice any of the following signs of too much exercise:

- Unusual or persistent fatigue

- Increased weakness

- Decreased range of motion

- Increased joint swelling

- Continuing pain (lasting for more than an hour after exercising)[22]

THE BENEFITS OF BEING PROACTIVE

As a physical therapist, Margrey has worked with many lupus patients over the years. She has observed that the people who do well with lupus in the long run (including her) are the ones who live independent and productive lives. They are the ones who have maintained their flexibility, their muscle strength, and aerobic capacity. And they are the ones who have stayed active with a positive attitude. "At the clinic I've seen what worse looks like," she says, "so I don't spend any time complaining or making excuses."

Margrey's observation that, in addition to exercise and diet, a positive attitude plays a large role in the management of lupus is right on track. Chapter 6 will give you more details about the power of the mind.

CHAPTER 6

The Mind-Body Relationship

⚏

You have a chronic illness that has changed your life. There is no cure and the medications prescribed to manage one problem usually cause other problems. You feel achy and tired on your good days and have no way of knowing when the disease will flare and send you to bed or even to the hospital. Are you unhappy about this?

This rhetorical question sounds a bit ridiculous to anyone with lupus. Of course it is very difficult, mentally and emotionally, to live with a chronic illness. This is not the life you had planned for yourself, yet it's the one you've got. But interestingly, although you may not be happy about having lupus, your ability to accept it, deal with it, and move on can greatly influence the severity of your symptoms and ultimately the quality of your life. This chapter takes a close-up look at the mind-body connection in lupus and offers you some tips for managing the mental and emotional aspects of this disease.

THE TRUTH ABOUT DEPRESSION AND LUPUS

Lupus and depression frequently go together, but unfortunately because the management of lupus can be so intense and time-consuming, the problems associated with depression are too frequently ignored or even left undiagnosed.

If you know you are suffering from both lupus and depression or if you have lupus and wonder if you might also have depression, medical advocates strongly urge you to see the two as separate medical entities and seek appropriate treatment for *both*—especially in view of the way each can influence the other:

- The depression caused by chronic illness often aggravates the illness; this is especially true in the case of lupus because it is well known that depression increases the perception of pain. It also causes fatigue and lethargy that can exacerbate the loss of energy caused by lupus.

- Depression impairs the immune system, which is especially problematic in an autoimmune disease like lupus. In one study, 42 young adults had blood tests that evaluated their immune function. Half were depressed, half were not. Compared with the normal participants, the depressed group showed significant immune impairment.[1]

- Depression can affect the dosing requirements of your medications. It can also put you at greater risk of experiencing side effects, which is already a major concern in the treatment of lupus.

- Depression robs you of the mental stamina you need to live with a chronic illness. You are less able to take control of your disease and improve the quality of your life.

If you are feeling depressed, don't lump the symptoms in with those of lupus. Depression is a highly treatable condition that you can do something about.

Symptoms of Depression

Depression frequently goes unnoticed in those with lupus because it presents similar symptoms. In SLE, symptoms such as lethargy, loss of energy and interest, insomnia, pain, and diminished sexual interest and performance are common and readily assigned to the disease without any thought given to the possibility that these same symptoms might be signs of depressive illness. In his article, "Depression in Lupus," Howard S. Shapiro, M.D., cautions, "Most cases of depressive illness go unrecognized and untreated until the later stages of the illness when the severity of the depression becomes unbearable to the patient, and/or until the family or physician can no longer ignore it. In fact, several studies indicate that between 30 and 50 percent of cases of major depressive illness go undiagnosed in medical settings. Perhaps more disturbing is that many studies indicate that major depressive disorders in the medically ill are undertreated and/or inadequately treated, even when recognized."[2]

In order to recognize and then do something about depression, you need to be able to identify its symptoms. First, keep in mind that depression isn't the same as sadness or a sense of feeling down or anxious. We all have those feelings at different times throughout our lives. Clinical depression makes it almost impossible to carry on usual activities, sleep, eat, or enjoy life. Pleasure seems a thing of the past. The National Institutes of Mental Health advice is that if you have experienced four or more of the following symptoms for more than 2 weeks, you are at risk for clinical depression and should have a physical and psychological evaluation by a medical physician:

- A persistent sad, anxious, or "empty" mood
- Loss of interest or pleasure in ordinary activities, including sex
- Sleep problems (insomnia, oversleeping, early-morning waking)
- Eating problems (loss of appetite or weight, weight gain)
- Difficulty concentrating, remembering, or making decisions
- Feelings of hopelessness or pessimism
- Feelings of guilt, worthlessness, or helplessness
- Thoughts of death or suicide; a suicide attempt
- Irritability
- Excessive crying
- Recurring aches and pains that don't respond to treatment[3]

Causes of Depression

If you have lupus and experience depression, it may be rooted in one or a combination of the following causes.

Lupus Itself

According to Drs. Lahita and Phillips in *Lupus: Everything You Need to Know*, depression can absolutely be the result of lupus. In fact, they say, "Some 67 percent of patients with lupus have psychological abnormalities. These range from neurotic problems to actual psychosis, and can often be related to central nervous system involvement."[4]

Medications

Many of the medications used in the treatment of lupus can cause side effects that alter mood and emotional control and may lead to depression. In his article, "Psychiatric Side Effects of Medicines Used in SLE," Howard Shapiro, M.D., states the following:

Learn More

Find out more about depression by contacting these organizations:

National Foundation for Depressive Illness
P.O. Box 2257
New York, NY 10116
Phone: (800) 239-1265
Web site: www.depression.org

National Mental Health Association
1021 Prince Street
Alexandria, VA 22314
Phone: (800) 969-6642
Web site: www.nmha.org

- Depression has been associated with some of the NSAIDs, especially with ibuprofen, fenoprofen, and naproxen.

- The antimalarial drugs, especially chloroquine, have been associated with a number of psychiatric reactions when taken in high doses. Generally speaking, the "mild side effects," such as tiredness and depression occur more frequently with chloroquine (40 percent) than with hydroxychloroquine (29 percent).

- By and large, the medical literature states that the most common side effect of steroids is depression. In general, steroid reactions occur soon after the drugs are started, primarily within the first few weeks.[5]

Life Changes Caused by Chronic Illness

Living with lupus can be an emotional struggle (especially when you "look fine"). If you feel somehow responsible for your illness, you may feel a sense of shame, worthlessness, or isolation. You may feel great uncertainty about your future. You may not be able to perform up to the level you're used to. Helen Grusd, Ph.D., a licensed clinical psychologist from Los Angeles, believes that you may need to mourn the death of your good health. "Just like you would mourn the loss of a loved one," she says, "you go through various stages of grief when your health is taken from you. You go through shock and disbelief. Then you go through a sadness and a rage. Then a time of bargaining ('If I take this health product and change my diet, will you let me beat this?'), and then eventually there is acceptance of the fact that this is a chronic illness and you won't have the kind of health you had before. But it takes time and often professional help to reach this stage."

> *You may need to mourn the death of your good health. Just like you would mourn the loss of a loved one, you go through various stages of grief when your health is taken from you.*
>
> —HELEN GRUSD, PH.D.

Something Unrelated to Lupus

It is common to attribute all physical and mental health problems to a chronic medical condition, but there is a possibility that even if you didn't have lupus, you might still suffer from a depressive illness rooted in some other cause.

"I don't believe it matters that much what causes the depression," says Dr. Grusd. "When people are depressed for any reason it affects their whole lives. It affects the course of their treatment; it affects their perception of life; and more important, it robs them of the feeling that they have some control over their lives and makes them feel helpless and hopeless. All of this can affect the course of the illness because it can lead to a perception of increased pain, more chronic fatigue, greater joint pain, and a generalized sense of not feeling well. I believe that if people could learn preventive coping skills that could help them learn how to deal with this new life, this could treat or even prevent depression."

Treatment of Depression

Serious depression is not something to be ignored because it will "probably go away on its own." It is a serious medical condition that needs prompt medical attention. Dr. Shapiro confidently states, "Clinical depression in the physically ill generally responds well to standard psychiatric treatments and so patients treated only for their physical illness will suffer needlessly the effects of clinical depression."[6] Don't ignore depression because you already have lupus—they both deserve your attention.

The first line of medical treatment for depression is often medication. Your physician may prescribe any number of specific psychopharmacological agents, such as minor tranquilizers, hypnotics, antianxiety agents, sedatives, various types of antidepressants, muscle relaxants, beta-blockers, and psychostimulants. If the physician who is treating your depression is not the doctor who is treating your lupus, be sure he or she knows your full medical history. Some of these medications are not safe for those with weakened liver or kidneys and some may interact with other medications you may be taking.

Along with medication, your physician will probably recommend some sort of psychological therapy and relaxation regimen. These are vital components of an effective program to treat depression. These give you the knowledge and the tools you'll need to be actively involved in your mind-body health. "The key," says Dr. Grusd, "is for the patient to feel empowered and involved in the treatment of the illness, and to participate actively in the healing process. This can be done by living consciously and being aware of one's thoughts, feelings, and belief systems, and rewriting life scripts that are sabotaging a more effective and meaningful life. By increasing the areas of their lives they do have control of, chronically ill patients can maximize their sense of well-being and efficacy, which can contribute to the relative improvement of their health. The challenge for the chronically ill is to revisit their mission statements, rewrite different relevant and exciting ones that are congruent with their values, beliefs, and changed lifestyles. Dealing with lupus or any chronic illness forces a person to answer questions such as, 'Who am I?' 'What is my purpose?' and 'Where am I going?' These are questions that healthy people should be asking as well, but they often don't, and only do so when they are compelled to by some crisis."

> *Dealing with lupus or any chronic illness forces a person to answer questions such as, "Who am I?" "What is my purpose?" and "Where am I going?"*
>
> —HELEN GRUSD, PH.D.

You can begin to treat or prevent serious depression by understanding the mind-body relationship and the kinds of psychological therapies and relaxation strategies that can be used to bring the two into harmony.

MIND-BODY THERAPY

Although there is no doubt that the pain and other symptoms of lupus are not just "all in your head," there is also no doubt that the way you think about having a chronic illness can affect the way you actually experience it. Medical professionals know that people's thoughts have a physical impact on the body.

For example, if you're having negative thoughts such as, "I'll never get better" or "This is ruining my life," that will impact your ability to cope emotionally with the disease. But these thoughts can also work against you on a very physical level. Negative thoughts begin a spiral of physical reactions that start in the brain and can lead to physical changes caused by stress. Sympathetic nervous system activity can be activated by negative thoughts to release chemicals such as adrenaline and the stress hormone cortisol; you can then experience rapid heart rate, muscle tension, and increased blood pressure, which can exacerbate your symptoms. (For details about the sympathetic nervous system and the stress reaction, see "The Effects of Stress and Lupus" beginning on page 171.)

Fortunately, you can interrupt this stress reaction if you intervene at the point where it begins—at the level of thought.

Cognitive-Behavioral Therapy

Many therapists use what's called cognitive-behavioral therapy (CBT) to help people with chronic illnesses live positive and fulfilling lives. CBT focuses on negative or noncoping thoughts and actions caused by things such as chronic illness, persistent pain, and repeated treatment failures. This therapy recognizes that total denial of a chronic illness allows the disease to progress unchecked and leads to long-term physical and psychological complications. On the other hand, this therapy also addresses the fact that when obsession with one's health allows the chronic illness to become a controlling life force, a great sense of helplessness and hopelessness can result, which drastically reduces one's quality of life. Cognitive-behavioral therapy turns that helplessness or denial around by giving you control. It teaches you that you are not a hapless victim. It shows you that the way you think about your illness, and therefore the way you act, can strongly influence the way you live with lupus.

Finding Acceptance with Cognitive-Behavioral Therapy

Cognitive-behavioral therapy requires you to use a rather simple two-step process:

1. Identify your negative or counterproductive thoughts.

2. Change those thoughts and the actions that follow them to a more positive direction.

"If, for example," says Katina Rodis, Ph.D., "you are in denial, your negative thought is the insistence that there's nothing wrong with you, you can do whatever you want, and you do not have to change your life at all. You do not have to take so many medications and you can go to the beach and sunbathe with your friends if you want. You need to reframe those thoughts and acknowledge, 'I now have a chronic illness and so my life will not be exactly like it was before. But my worth does not depend on what or how much I do. I can help myself feel better and lead a good life if I follow doctor's orders, stay out of the sun, and take it easy today.'"

Once the negative thoughts are identified and countered, they need to be followed by a positive action. You might, for example, do what Dr. Rodis does to deal with chronic fatigue. "I've learned to make a list of all the things I plan to do each day and then eliminate 50 percent of those plans," she says. This 50-percent solution is a realistic way of training yourself to accept your new life and set priorities. Cognitive-behavioral therapy

> *You need to reframe denial and negativity by acknowledging, "I now have a chronic illness, my life won't be exactly like it was before. But my worth doesn't depend on what or how much I do."*
>
> —KATINA RODIS, PH.D.

Searching for an Identity Beyond Lupus

Katina Rodis, Ph.D., a clinical psychologist from Concord, Massachusetts, has had systemic lupus erythematosus with kidney and central nervous system involvement for 21 years. "At age 30, just as I began working as a licensed therapist in a psychiatric hospital," remembers Dr. Rodis, "I found I was feeling exhausted all the time. Here I was working with high-intensity psychiatric emergencies and I was falling asleep at my desk. I went to my therapist and wondered out loud if maybe the fatigue was caused by depression." Dr. Rodis' therapist suggested she have a complete medical checkup, which she did. The various blood tests showed many abnormalities, but no one identified the patterns common in lupus and so it took quite a long time to get a correct diagnosis. "There was still a lot of controversy at that time about whether or not lupus was in fact a real illness or some kind of garbage pail category. But I continued to get worse and when I finally became very ill (and just barely escaped brain surgery for a misdiagnosed pituitary adenoma) I finally got a diagnosis of lupus."

Life from then on was quite different for Dr. Rodis. "I tried very hard to hold on to the life I had, but I was very sick for many years and eventually I had to give up work. I took me a long time to ac-

asks you to ask yourself: What is really important to me and what can I do without risking a flare and further illness? "You can discover some very wonderful things about yourself," says Dr. Rodis, "if you allow yourself to live with the disease rather than trying to rail against it. Being angry because you have lupus is a waste of precious energy that gets you nowhere."

Dr. Rodis knows it isn't easy to consistently use cognitive-behavioral restructuring, especially because the rewards of positive and constructive thinking are not immediate. "You could be thinking and doing all the right things and still have a flare anyway. This makes it hard to keep cept that I needed to make some radical modifications in my life if I was going to live well with this disease. The problem that I have had, and the problem with many of the people I have treated, is the fact that in most cases lupus occurs in adulthood. This happens after we have created an image of ourselves as a well person who can do certain things. (I, for example, rode horses!) Now we have to completely revamp that image, which is very difficult. I remember struggling with identity issues such as: If I'm not a working therapist, what am I? If I accept Social Security money, am I a parasite on society? We are in a society that defines itself by what people do, not who they are. This was difficult for me to get over."

The problem of accepting lupus as a chronic illness is compounded by the fact that the symptoms go into remission for a while and give you the feeling that you're well again. "The tendency is to want to slip into denial immediately and take on the role of the old healthy self that we didn't want to give up in the first place," says Dr. Rodis. "Then comes the relapse and we go through the emotional assault all over again. It is far better to learn how to reposition yourself in the world than to live for moments of remission and crash in times of relapse."

doing the things you've been told are good for you. I have a lot of sympathy for this in my own life, but deep down I know that pushing too hard and denying that I have a chronic illness never works out for me in the long run. And so I keep trying to accept my limitations."

Breaking Negative Patterns with Cognitive-Behavioral Therapy

On the flip side of those who try to deny having lupus are those who use their illness unconsciously to gain some secondary benefit. In this case, cognitive-behavior therapy can be used to break negative patterns such as excessive use of drugs, avoidance of activity, and dependence on others. This therapy encourages and rewards the very opposite of these behaviors: responsibility, independence, activity, and the desire to free oneself from the disease rather than be bound to it.

This all begins with the way you talk to yourself. When you start to pay attention to what you think and say about your illness, you might hear yourself making comments such as, "Oh, my aching joints." Then notice what you decide to do about that thought. Will you stay home from work? Reach for more medication? Or, decide to get back into bed and wait for the pain or fatigue to ease. If the consequences of these behaviors are positive, the behavior will increase in occurrence. If, for example, you get attention when you complain, you'll continue to complain. If you can avoid doing an unpleasant task because you are in pain, you might find yourself more aware of your pain. It's not just you—we're all like that. We repeat thoughts and actions that give us some kind of personal benefit. To find out if you may need to do some cognitive and behavioral restructuring, ask yourself the following questions:

- Do I avoid physical activity to "protect" myself?

- Have I stopped socializing because of my illness?

- Do I want others to take care of me?

- Do I rely on excessive medication to control my illness?

> You have a physical illness that has a physical base to it, but you can develop behaviors based on the way you think about it.

- Do I often groan, limp, rub, brace myself, or talk about my illness and pain?

- Do I get attention by talking about my illness?

- Do I use my illness to avoid undesirable activities?

- Do I sustain my illness in the hope of gaining monetary compensation?

These questions are not insulting—they simply require an honest reevaluation of how you may be reacting to a very difficult chronic illness. You have a physical illness that has a physical base to it, but you can develop behaviors based on the way you think about and react to your situation. Identifying these behaviors will not get rid of your disease or your pain—the symptoms of lupus are very real—but you have a choice about how you react to them.

Changing the Way You Think About Lupus

Cognitive therapy will help you recognize your own self-talk attitudes and identify the statements you say to yourself that are making it harder than necessary for you to live with a chronic condition. For people living with lupus, it's vital to disease management to understand the clear relationship between the way you think about your health and the way you feel it. For this reason, cognitive-behavioral therapy definitely belongs in your treatment program for lupus.

For some people, CBT is best learned and practiced under the guidance and supervision of a trained therapist. Other people may find better support through close friends, family, and support-group members. Either way, with some persistence and practice you can learn to identify your negative thoughts and behaviors, challenge them, and replace them with more appropriate thoughts and actions. When you learn to change the way you think about your illness and the way you act in response to those thoughts, you have a powerful mind-body tool that will help you lead a productive and positive life. This therapy can also help you learn, as Dr. Rodis says, "Lupus is not your enemy. It's just part of who you are now. You can still create a life that is full and good, even though you can't always do what you used to do." You may not have the same life you had before lupus, but it's the only one you have, so when you talk to yourself, be kind and encouraging.

> *Lupus is not your enemy. It's just part of who you are now. You can still create a life that is full and good, even though you can't always do what you used to do.*
>
> —KATINA RODIS, PH.D.

Interrupt Negative Thoughts and
Practice Positive Thoughts

Starting today, put cognitive-behavioral therapy into action. Recognize and interrupt negative thoughts and then replace them with positive thoughts. What follows will show you how easy this can be if you give it a good try.

Interrupt Negative Thoughts

When you talk to yourself, what do you say? Stop the thought immediately if you hear yourself getting wrapped up in any of these negative patterns:

Catastrophizing	"My life is ruined."
Overgeneralizing	"This will never end."
Personalizing	"Leave it to me to have this kind of pain."
Obsessing	"This is awful. This is terrible. I can't stand this."

Practice Positive Thoughts

You can use kind affirmations to restructure the way you talk to yourself. Instead of kicking yourself and saying things like, "I'm so pathetic," or "How could anybody love me?" be kind to yourself with loving words. Make a habit of saying things like:

"It takes a courageous person to live with this illness."

"I love and believe in myself."

"I'm learning how to take control of this illness and live a good life."

"I accept myself the way I am and will make the best of this life I have."

"I am a good person."

THE EFFECTS OF STRESS ON LUPUS

Research strongly supports what you probably already know: Stress aggravates the symptoms of lupus. What happens physically in your body during periods of stress is really quite dramatic and has the power to make you feel absolutely miserable. Here's why.

The roots of the body's physical response to stress go back to our primitive days. In the era of the caveman, the difference between bringing an animal home to eat and being eaten by the animal was a person's ability to react quickly to danger. The human body had to be able to prepare for "fight or flight" at a moment's notice. To do this, the sympathetic portion of the autonomic nervous system of the body sent out norepinephrine neurons, which influence all major organs and cause the adrenal glands to release adrenaline (epinephrine). Adrenaline causes rapid heart rate, dry mouth, increased blood pressure, dilated pupils, sweating, the redirection of blood flow to the muscles and away from the digestive tract and skin (causing the pale look of terror), and muscle tremor.

The problem is that this stress response, which was designed to promote the physical activity of running away or fighting, is rarely appropriate for us today. When we are stuck in traffic and late for an appointment, we do not need extra oxygen directed to our deep muscles, and yet it happens. Even with no foe in sight and nowhere to run, our heart beats rapidly, our blood pressure rises, and our muscles tighten.

> *The problem is that this stress response, which was designed to promote the physical activity of running away or fighting, is rarely appropriate for us today.*

To add to this bodily assault, during the stress response a complex process causes the release of the stress hormone cortisol into the bloodstream. Cortisol can cause a simple stressful situation to have negative consequences on the body lasting from several hours to weeks and months if the stress is repeated and chronic (such as the stress you feel when you have to deal with persistent joint pain).

Initially, the cortisol released during stress has several good purposes. It suppresses the immune system, which, if you are in a fight (or running from a predator), keeps a small injury from swelling up and interfering with your ability to fight back or get away. Cortisol also causes the level of blood sugar to rise, making it more available for use in the brain and muscles for energy and quick action. Cortisol reaches the brain and acutely acts as a stimulant, heightening your sense of awareness.

In the long run, however, the release of cortisol in severe or chronic stress will take an undesirable toll on the body. In animals, the long-term exposure to stress beyond the animal's control or in a repeated fashion, results in a depression-like syndrome called "learned helplessness." In this state, the animal loses drive, interacts less with other animals, becomes slower in movement, and eventually even dies. In the brains of such animals, release of cortisol becomes continuous. Neurons that release cortisol remain activated for extended periods, causing burnout or depression.[7]

The constant release of adrenaline and cortisol that's caused by unrelenting stress of both daily life and chronic illness fuels the symptoms of lupus. Letting stress go unchecked is like supercharging your lupus. That's why relaxation techniques are an important part of any treatment program for this disease.

The most direct way in which stress affects the pain of lupus is through the instinctive reaction to guard and brace. We tense up our muscles and hold our bodies in certain postures, which does sometimes give some relief in a specific area, but causes bigger problems in the long run. Chronic pain conditions tend to lead to chronic muscle tension. This causes the muscles to use more energy and become fatigued—both of which add to the level of pain—creating a vicious cycle. Also, the longer you tense up, the more likely you are to cause the muscles to actually shorten and cut down on your range of motion and flexibility.

In addition to the muscle tension caused by the guard-and-brace reaction to pain, people with lupus are also subject to the same daily

The Power of Relaxation

Reducing stress reduces the symptoms of lupus in a number of ways:

- Relaxation exercises can control the involuntary workings of the nervous system that are known to support and aggravate pain. These techniques can help you manage pain by influencing blood pressure, heart rate, respiration, and metabolism—all seemingly involuntary physiological functions that power the chronic pain cycle.

- Relaxation exercises enhance the quality of sleep. Relaxation techniques calm the body, improve circulation, and lower anxiety levels—all of which promote peaceful rest.

- Relaxation therapy reduces the sensation of pain by decreasing muscle tension.

- Relaxation techniques reduce anxiety. It's difficult to think positively and continue your pain-management regimen each day if you are chronically anxious and tense.

- Relaxation exercises improve your sense of control over pain. They put you in charge; they give you an active role in managing your pain. This reduces the feelings of helplessness and hopelessness that support and maintain pain.

tensions as everyone else, which adds to muscle tension. If you are treated rudely by a customer service rep on the telephone and find your heart pounding and your blood pressure rising, you are further aggravating an already difficult medical condition. This is wasted energy that people with lupus can't afford to give away. But a person who knows how to use some simple relaxation techniques could use that circumstance as an opportunity to increase body energy and ease pain.

LEARNING TO RELAX

To use relaxation techniques most effectively, you have to begin to listen to your body and understand how, where, and when you hold on to tension. You have to know that a trip to the dentist can throw you into a lupus flare if you're the kind of patient who grips your seat and tenses your entire body while in the dentist's chair. You have to learn to recognize what muscle tension feels like and then learn how to relax.

But deciding to "relax" is easier said than done. Relaxation is a skill just like any other skill that needs time and practice to perfect—but don't turn it into a chore. When you use the relaxation techniques explained in this section, do them in ways that are easy and, of course, "relaxing." You defeat the purpose if you begin by thinking, "I have to put aside 45 minutes tonight to relax," or "I have to make time to follow this hour-long relaxation tape and do all the things it tells me." Even if you make it through a few sessions, the demanding schedule will soon make you decide that relaxation just isn't for you.

The rest of the chapter is devoted to relaxation techniques that you can learn to change the way your body handles the stress of lupus and everyday life. In this section you'll learn the value of deep breathing, mental imagery, progressive muscle relaxation, aromatherapy, biofeedback, and hypnosis.

Deep Breathing

People with lupus (as well as many other people in stressful situations) tend to breathe with their chest muscles. If you take a deep breath right now, you may find that your chest puffs out as you fill your lungs with air. This breathing habit is adding to your pain and fatigue! Watch a child as he sleeps and you'll see the stomach muscles rise up with each breath as the diaphragm, not the chest, fills with air. Many adults have lost this natural deep-breathing mechanism that is most efficient in bringing restorative oxygen to all tissues of the body.

Every day, practice breathing from your diaphragm:

1. Place one hand on your chest and the other on your stomach.

2. As you take a deep breath in, feel the hand on your stomach rise. The hand on your chest should not rise.

3. Let the air go. Don't push it out. Let it go gently. Feel the hand on your stomach go down.

When you have the knack of diaphragm breathing, focus on the pace of your breathing. Short, shallow breaths are stressful to the body. As you practice this deep-breathing technique, change your pace to six breaths per minute. (If you check your "natural" breathing pattern right now, you may find that you're taking about 10 breaths per minute.) Take in a slow, easy breath to the count of 4. Then release the breath to the count of 4. Hold your breath for 2 seconds. This 10-second cycle will give you 6 breaths per minute.

Deep breathing is a strategy you can use anywhere. No one around you needs to know you're practicing a stress-reduction technique. It's a technique you can engage in whenever you feel your pain increasing and your body tensing. Automatically, deep breathing will change your body's stress reaction.

In the beginning, you'll find that although the deep-breathing exercise is easy, your chest-breathing habit will return as soon as you're not paying attention. Give yourself a couple of weeks of practicing deep breathing just a few minutes here and there throughout the day and soon you'll find that your body will relearn how to breathe correctly on its own.

Mental Imagery

In order to feel pain, your brain has to perceive it. Mental imagery literally takes your mind off your pain and focuses it on something positive, which causes the brain to release brain chemicals that elevate mood and diminish pain—really!

The goal with mental imagery for relaxation is to ease the muscle tension of stress by tricking the body into thinking you're relaxed and having a good time. Sit back, close your eyes, and imagine a very pleasant incident or place. For example, some people find this kind of image soothing:

> I am stretched out on the ocean beach. The sun is warm on my body. When it gets too strong, I have an umbrella for protection. I feel the warmth of the sand on my fingertips. I see the calm ocean touching the shore. I can smell the salt of the ocean, and I can taste the sea air. On my beach there are just the right number of people—I'm not crowded or lonely. On my beach there are no sand crabs or flies. I feel just wonderful. It's an ideal place that I can visit with all my senses anytime I want. Even when I'm in the middle of a crowd with my eyes wide open, I can go to my beach.

This safe, pleasant place happens to be a beach—yours can be anywhere. It can be in your family room by the fireplace, the woods by a stream, the park down the street. Here are some points to consider in creating and visiting your safe place:

- Make the place real. When you're stressed or in pain, you won't be able to relate to an alien planet.

- Involve all of your senses. Make sure all the smells and the things you touch, taste, hear, and see in this environment are pleasing to you.

- Go to this place often. The more you practice increasing the quality of your image, the more you can rely on it when you're in pain. It will become a practiced response.

Progressive Muscle Relaxation

In stressful situations, many people describe the way they feel as being "tied up in knots." Due to the way our muscles react to stress, this actually is true. Progressive muscle relaxation will help you untie the knots by teaching you how to recognize muscle tension and then how to relax the involved muscles. Then when you feel stress from physical pain, you can relax those muscles that are aggravating your pain. By practicing progressive muscle relaxation, you will learn what it feels like when stress begins to manifest itself in muscle tension. Then when your muscles do begin to tense involuntarily, you will be able to identify the problem area and stop the stress attack.

To begin, get yourself into a comfortable position. Sit back in a large cushioned chair or lie down on a couch or bed. Then go through your body and tense and relax one muscle muscle group at a time. Let's start with your right hand and arm. Clench your hand into a tight fist and tightly tense the muscles in your lower arm. Feel where the tension goes from your hand, up your arm, into your shoulder, right into your neck. Maintain that tension for 5 to 10 seconds so you have time to feel how whole parts of your body are involved in tension. Then relax. Feel the experience of letting go, of consciously relaxing your muscles.

> *By practicing progressive muscle relaxation, you will learn what it feels like when stress begins to manifest itself in muscle tension.*

Then move to the other arm, then to other muscle groups: Do this exercise with each leg and foot; the abdomen and chest; and the face, jaw, and forehead.

By repeating this exercise, muscle group by muscle group throughout the body, you develop more and more control over the muscles and become increasingly sensitive and attuned to how a tense muscle and a relaxed muscle feel. Frequent repetition of short practice times throughout the day is a good way to learn this skill.

Other Relaxation Strategies

When you're comfortable with these basics, go on to explore other types of relaxation strategies. There is no strategy created specifically for lupus; anything you find that leads you to a relaxed state will improve your overall pain state. You can find books on various relaxation programs in your library or bookstore. (The classic in this field is Dr. Herbert Benson's *The Relaxation Response*.) You can buy relaxation audio and videotapes that walk you through the steps of various relaxation exercises. Or you can sign up to take a class in more advanced types of relaxation techniques, such as yoga and meditation, which may require some guidance and supervision to use them effectively. A few you might want to explore are aromatherapy, biofeedback, and hypnosis.

Aromatherapy

Aromatherapy is a healing treatment that utilizes the essential oils of both cultivated and wild plants that emit an aroma as they evaporate. Essential oils are found in the petals (lavender), leaves (basil), wood (cedarwood), fruit (orange), seeds (sesame), roots (ginger), gum (myrrh), and resin (pine) of plants and trees. In many cases, the oils are located in more than one part of the plant or tree. Orange, for example, has essential oils in the rind of the fruit, as well as the white flowers and leaves of the tree.

Two plants in particular (lavender and rosemary) have been found to affect mood and state of mind and can be used as a form of relaxation therapy.

Two plants in particular have been found to affect mood and state of mind and can be used as a form of relaxation therapy. A study at the University of Miami Medical School found that people who inhaled the scent of lavender or rosemary were less anxious and more relaxed. Participants in the lavender group experienced an increase in beta-band activity (suggesting drowsiness), an improvement in mood, and a feeling of greater relaxation. The rosemary group showed a decrease in alpha and beta activity, suggesting alertness and lower levels of anxiety.[8] Other oils with calming properties include chamomile, geranium, and neroli.

Since it is safe and inexpensive, you might want to make aromatherapy a part of your relaxation regimen. According to Myra Cameron, author of *Mother Nature's Guide to Vibrant Beauty and Health*, you can do this in three ways: inhalation, water therapy, or massage. She explains, "Whether in mist or liquid form, essential oils are able to penetrate easily through the skin due to their small molecules. This sounds surprising because usually oils have large molecules that sit on the surface of the skin. But essential oils do not have an oily texture. Actually, they are the complete opposite of oils because they are not heavy or greasy. These oils are called 'volatile' liquids because they evaporate when exposed to the air. They feel as light to the touch as water or alcohol. They disappear almost instantly when applied to the skin."[9]

Try inhalation, water therapy, and massage according to the following instructions offered by Cameron and you'll soon find that this relaxation exercise is something you look forward to at the end of a long day.[10]

Inhalation

Breathing in droplets of an essential oil brings its healing and soothing powers directly into your body. There are a number of ways to mist the air:

Steam. Add 6 to 12 drops of the selected oil to a bowl of steaming hot water. Place a towel over your head and breathe deeply.

Fragrancer. These attractive pots are easy to use. Fill the top bowl with water and add 3 to 6 drops of the essential oil on the surface. The candle in the pot underneath heats the water, slowly releasing the natural fragrance of the oil into the room.

Diffuser. You can buy an electric diffuser that gently mists the essential oil into the air.

Humidifier. You can add an essential oil to the water of a humidifier to mist the air. Or you can simply add a few drops of oil to a small bowl of water and place it on top of a radiator.

Lightbulb. You can disperse an essential oil into the air by placing a few drops of the oil on a lightbulb. Place 2 or 3 drops on the bulb while it is still cold. (Never place it on a hot lightbulb.) As the bulb heats up, it will speed up the evaporation process and fill the room with fragrance.

Handkerchief. Add 3 or 4 drops of an essential oil to a handkerchief. Place the handkerchief close to your nose and inhale. This is especially useful when you are on the go to help calm nerves or clear congestion.

Water Therapy

The calming power of water has been utilized to soothe life's tensions for centuries. Here are a few ways to combine water therapy with aromatherapy for a relaxing retreat:

Bath. Taking a bath mixed with an essential oil is a wonderful way to combine skin penetration and inhalation. Don't run an extremely hot bath. Lukewarm water is the best temperature for therapeutic value; because the water is close to your body's temperature, it produces a relaxing and soothing action. Add 5 to 10 drops of the essential oil to the bath while the water is running. Before you enter the tub, swish the water around so the essential oils mix well with the water. (Essential oils can mark plastic baths if they are not dispersed thoroughly.) If you have dry or sensitive skin, mix the essential oils with 1 ounce of a carrier oil such as sweet almond oil, wheat-germ oil, or macadamia nut oil. Then add this mixture to the bath and swish to mix. Now lie back in the water and breathe in deeply to inhale the oil vapor evaporating and rising from the oil droplets in the bath water. At the same time, relax and let your body absorb the oil through your skin.

> *The calming power of water has been utilized to soothe life's tensions for centuries.*

Shower. You can use essential oils in your shower, too. After washing and rinsing your body, dip a wet sponge in an oil mix of your choice and squeeze and rub this over your whole body while under a warm shower spray.

Footbath. Add a few drops of lavender oil to a bowl of hot water and soak your feet.

Sauna. Add 2 drops of an essential oil to a half-pint of water. Throw the water over the hot coals in the sauna to evaporate.

Massage

As a therapy in its own right, massage is a great way to beat stress, promote relaxation, relieve muscle tension and stiffness, and encourage better circulation. On a mental level, massage can promote a calm state of mind, increase alertness, and reduce mental stress. When you add aromatherapy to this form of care, your mind and body will also respond to the therapeutic action of the oil. (A partner is helpful for massaging hard-to-reach places, but you can massage essential oils into your skin for their soothing properties.)

As a therapy in its own right, massage is a great way to beat stress, promote relaxation, relieve muscle tension and stiffness, and encourage better circulation.

The following are useful tips for using essential oils in massage:

- Do not apply an essential oil directly to the skin (unless directed by an experienced aromatherapist) because it could cause an irritation.

- Mix and dilute essential oils with what is called a *carrier* or *base* oil. Some excellent oils for this purpose are almond oil, macadamia nut oil, and apricot kernel oil.

- Before applying the oil, warm it in your hands so that it is slightly warm when applied to the skin.

- Avoid showering for up to 3 to 4 hours after an essential oil massage because you don't want to rinse away the therapeutic value of the oils.

Used medicinally over the centuries, essential oils are now finding their way back into the family medicine cabinet and can be purchased in health food stores, herbal shops, and in bath and beauty shops. Risks are essentially nonexistent, and the cost is low.

Biofeedback

People are quick to say, "Oh, just relax!" But the truth is that it is a rare person who can truly tell when his or her body is tense. That's why many people with lupus find biofeedback very helpful.

The Association of Applied Psychophysiology and Biofeedback tells us, "The word 'biofeedback' was coined in 1969 to describe laboratory procedures (developed in the 1940s) that trained research subjects to alter brain activity, blood pressure, muscle tension, heart rate, and other bodily functions that are not normally controlled voluntarily. Biofeedback is a training technique in which people are taught to improve their health and performance by using signals from their own bodies."[11]

One commonly used device, for example, picks up electrical signals from the muscles. Every time muscles become tense this device triggers a flashing light or activates a beeper. If you want to slow down the flashing or beeping, you must lean how to relax the tense muscles. After you learn to control muscle tension, you can shake off the effects of stress anywhere, anytime without being attached to the sensors. Other biological functions that are commonly measured and used in a similar way to help people learn to control their physical functioning are skin temperature, heart rate, sweat gland activity, and brainwave activity. Studies have shown that we have more control over so-called involuntary bodily functions than we once thought possible.[12] What this means is that biofeedback helps you "see" your muscle tension and "see" how relaxation exercises can reduce the tension that contributes to your pain.

Resource Referral

To find a biofeedback practitioner near you, call the **Association of Applied Psychophysiology and Biofeedback (AAPB)** in Wheat Ridge, Colorado, at (303) 422-8436 or contact them through their Web site at www.aapb.org.

Hypnosis

Hypnosis is a state of deep relaxation in which the subconscious mind is extraordinarily receptive to positive thoughts and suggestions. When falling into a hypnotic trance, the brain follows the same steps apparent when falling to sleep. It is like descending a staircase with each step dropping you into a deeper state of relaxation. You begin with alpha brain waves, which are associated with relaxed wakefulness. Within minutes, these are replaced by slower, more regular theta waves. In this state, the body temperature begins to drop and the muscles relax. Here you can reach the hypnotic state. In 5 to 15 minutes of hypnotic trance at this stage of consciousness, a very tired and tense body moves into a relaxed state, as if you just had 8 hours of sleep.

Self-hypnosis is something that's definitely worth learning how to do, according to Katherine Fox, a board-certified clinical hypnotherapist in Davis, California. Fox herself has three autoimmune diseases (CREST [a benign form of scleroderma], Raynaud's phenomenon, and Sjögren's syndrome) and is absolutely sure that hypnosis offers a form of relaxation that can ease the tension of living with lupus and can even contribute to remission of symptoms.

"My favorite story that illustrates what hypnosis can do for someone with lupus," says Fox, "is one in which I had a female client, whose lupus was out of control, go into a complete remission. I helped this woman go into a hypnotic trance and mentally picture the lupus inside her body. She visualized her lupus as millions of shiny black disks in her bloodstream. Then I suggested that she mentally gather them all into the palm of her hand and throw them away—and to picture herself feeling better as she got rid of them." Fox then taught her client how to hypnotize herself and told her to keep mentally "checking inside" herself daily and to continue visualizing removing these black disks.

"When you get a diagnosis of lupus, it's intangible," says Fox. "You can't 'see' what the disease is. By visualizing lupus, it empowers you to help control your disease, and the relaxed state brought on by the hypnosis gives your body the strength it needs to fight back." Six years later, Fox reports, the woman's lupus remains in remission. "This isn't surprising," says Fox. "When I'm relaxed, I have very few symptoms of my autoimmune diseases, but when I've got too much going on and let my body get stressed, that's when I have trouble. Relaxation is part of the formula for remaining healthy; there is definitely a mind-body connection there."

Finding a Trained Hypnotherapist

Everyone is capable of self-hypnosis (as explained below) and need not rely on a trained hypnotherapist, but it's a good idea to have at least one session with a certified therapist to get you started. But be careful: Anyone can hang out a shingle and claim to be a hypnotist. As Fox explains, "It is my understanding that, to date, in most of the United States there are no laws or legislation governing hypnotherapists." But that doesn't mean you have to take anyone you find in the phone book. There are legitimate training schools and professional certifications for this type of therapy. According to Fox, training is based on hours. The initial 100 hours, level one, certifies you as a master hypnotist. This training gives an overview and foundation of hypnosis. The second level, another 50 hours, certifies you as a hypnotherapist, which gives you in-depth training in all of the uses of hypnosis. And the third level, another 50 hours, certifies you as a clinical hypnotherapist, which is advance training in the field.

When you begin your search for a hypnotherapist, look for initials such as:

- C.H.T. (Certified Hypnotherapist)
- C.C.H.T. (Certified Clinical Hypnotherapist)
- Ct.H.A. (Certified Hypno-Anesthesiologist)

Fox suggests asking the following questions when looking for a hypnotherapist:

Finding a Hypnotherapist

You can find a certified hypnotherapist by contacting these organizations:

National Guild of Hypnotists
3 Lesa Drive
Merrimack, NH 03054
Phone: (603) 429-9438
Web site: www.ngh.net

American Board of Hypnotherapy
2002 E. McFadden Avenue
Santa Ana, CA 92705
Phone: (714) 245-9340 or (800) 872-9996
E-mail: aih@hypnosis.com
Web site: www.hypnosis.com/abh/abh.html

- How long have they been in practice? How long at their current location?

- Where were they trained? How many hours? Level of training? Other education?

- Are they members of any hypnotherapy association?

- What is their success rate?

- Do they belong to any local community associations, such as the Chamber of Commerce?

- Do they specialize in a certain area of hypnosis (weight loss, insomnia, relaxation, and so on)?

- Do they have any clients that you may call?

- What does a session cost?

- What is a typical session like? Will you be hypnotized in that first session?

Ask yourself:

- Does the therapist seem friendly, patient, and willing to answer my questions?

Self-Hypnosis

"The goal," says Fox, "is eventually to be able to use self-hypnosis any time, place, or situation—even at work or in a crowded football stadium—to calm down the body when you begin to feel stress. All it takes is the three main components of hypnosis, which are relaxation, concentration, and autosuggestion. You can learn all about these by reading books on the subject or listening to tapes that are available." According to Fox, the basic method of self-hypnosis follows these steps:

1. Sit down in a comfortable position and quietly begin repeating to yourself a word, a phrase, or what some call a mantra that is soothing to you.

2. Take three slow, deep breaths. The first is to relax yourself. The second is to move into a state of hypnosis and deeper relaxation. And the third is to *be* in a state of hypnosis.

3. Tell yourself how long you are going to be "in" hypnosis (for example, 10 or 15 minutes). This teaches you to set your inner clock.

4. Now start either at the tips of your toes or at the top of your head and move through each part of your body, relaxing the muscles and releasing all stress, anxiety, frustration. Say to yourself: "relax," "let go," "deeper and deeper."

5. Then imagine a staircase with ten steps or a path that will lead you to your "special place." Begin to count from ten down to one. On one, you will move into that special place in your mind. Spend a few minutes there, feeling, smelling, seeing, and hearing this special place.

If, for instance, you chose the beach—*hear* the waves, *smell* and *taste* the salty sea mist, *feel* the warmth of the sand between your toes, be completely relaxed at this beach. Or choose a mountain spot, a meadow, or anywhere you can feel safe and special.

6. Now begin your self-talk of positive suggestions and imagery. This is when you might imagine your lupus as a tangible object you can remove from your body. Or you can use self-affirming statements such as "I am learning to live well despite having lupus." Or, you can simply tell your body to relax and let go of all stress and tension.

7. To bring yourself out of a hypnotic trance, count up from one to five, suggesting that you have enjoyed a wonderful time of relaxation and on the count of five you will be back in your own body in the present time and will feel refreshed. Open your eyes, take a deep energizing breath, and stretch!

Self-hypnosis takes practice and focus, but it works. Don't let anyone tell you that hypnosis is nothing more than hocus pocus—it is a natural state of being that offers the potential for great physical and mental benefit with no risks and no side effects. It's certainly worth a try. For more information on hypnosis, go to Fox's Web site at www.hypnotherapy.net.

STRESS ALERT

While you're learning to recognize and release the body's negative physical responses to stress, you should also help your body avoid this tension to begin with by learning to reduce the amount of stress you expose yourself to each day. No one can eliminate stress completely (and who would want to live such a boring life!), but you can be on the alert for situations and people who tend to fill you with stress. If you know that a trip to the amusement park with your kids and their four friends will push you over the edge, don't go! If you know that a coworker's constant complaining and negative attitude make you feel tense, avoid her! If your job is so hectic and pressured that you feel you're about to explode every day of your life, think seriously about finding another job.

As someone with lupus, the quality of your daily life can be severely affected by the amount of stress with which you have to contend. So take an inventory of where excessive stress may be coming from and do something to change the situation. This is one area of your treatment plan that you have the power to control. Take a deep breath right now and promise yourself that you are going to do yourself the favor of avoiding stressful people and places. The next chapter will help you further improve the quality of your life as you come to understand better the way this illness affects your family, your career, and even your relationship with yourself.

CHAPTER 7

Living Well with Lupus

$\mathscr{O}$

AFTER YOU HAVE armed yourself with information about the symptoms, diagnosis, and treatment of lupus, life goes on. But what kind of life will that be? To live well with lupus you'll need to jump one more hurdle, the one built on the many relationships you've established in your life. Everyone around you is affected by your health. Your spouse (significant other, boyfriend or girlfriend), your children, your friends, coworkers, and employers all have to live with the reality that your chronic health condition affects the way you function, the way you feel physically and emotionally from one day to the next, and the way you relate to each one of them.

This chapter discusses how lupus affects your family life, your sex life, a pregnancy, and your career. It also explores how support groups can help you better live with your chronic illness.

FAMILY LIFE

Lupus can be tough on the whole family. This is especially true if the relationships were formed during a time of good health. If you married or built a life with a significant other before lupus, you established a relationship based on the assumption that you would be a happy, healthy life partner, but now that has changed. Your illness requires everyone to rethink daily responsibilities, and sometimes this leads to resentment and anger. Maybe you used to do most of the daily chores and child-care tasks, and now you need more help. Maybe you used to do the grocery shopping and wash the dishes, and now the shelves are often bare and the dishes are piled up in the sink. The anger, resentment, and guilt that these kinds of changes can cause can throw a relationship into a tailspin from which it can be hard to recover.

That's why you cannot ignore what's going on in your family and focus only on your symptoms and medical treatments. There's no doubt that the way your family lives with your lupus will have a strong effect on how you live with it, too.

Look at Both Sides of the Relationship

Getting on the right path is an important first step in finding a way to live with lupus. No one knows this better than Penney Cowan, the executive director of the American Chronic Pain Association (ACPA) in Rocklin, California. She has had fibromyalgia for 27 years and knows what it is like to live with a chronic pain and fatigue condition. In *American Chronic Pain Association Family Manual*, Cowan says, "Consider the family where one person has been forced to reduce activity levels, working hours, and financial responsibility. Suddenly the burden of supporting the family financially, emotionally, and physically falls on the well spouse. What are the chances of this family surviving long term if they cannot communicate their needs and feelings?"[1] We all know the odds are low. The person who can no longer do what he or she used to do feels frustrated, angry, and left out of the fun. The person who has to pick up the slack may feel let down, abused, and neglected. Children may feel afraid or even to blame.

Before writing the manual, Cowan interviewed families over a 3-year period. Her findings have helped her work with both the people in chronic pain and the families they live with. "The family members are usually the forgotten ones," says Cowan. "I found that they suffer in very much the same way except for the physical symptoms. All the painful emotions, the lost plans and dreams, the anger and frustration are theirs, too." Cowan believes that very often people with chronic conditions like lupus don't realize that their loved ones are also struggling and that's why they can't always be as supportive as they'd like to be.

Everyone in the family needs to learn how to acknowledge and communicate their emotional feelings. Everyone needs to be assertive and express personal feelings. When you're angry, frustrated, or happy, you have to be able to say so. Everyone in the family needs to know what's going on with everyone else. Living with someone who has a chronic condition is difficult—there's no point in trying to hide that—and so often family members hold all their feelings inside until they build up to the exploding point.

Once you realize that you are not the only one suffering from the effects of lupus, you can change the way you communicate with others. "Both sides need to acknowledge and validate that there are in fact real problems," says Cowan, "whether that's the pain and fatigue itself or the stress and confusion it causes. It's amazing how many walls can be quickly ripped down when people stop to acknowledge how another person is feeling and that both the person with lupus and his or her loved ones have problems to deal with." Cowan understands that it may be hard for you to feel empathy for your spouse who complains about having to do housework when you would love to do it if only your fatigue would lift or your pain would stop screaming for attention, but she says it's important to listen to your spouse's feelings without feeling personally criticized.

> *It's amazing how many walls can be quickly ripped down when people stop to acknowledge how another person is feeling and that both the person with lupus and his or her loved ones have problems to deal with.*
>
> —PENNEY COWAN

A sample conversation of validation that you might try with your family members could begin something like this: "I feel very bad that

I can't do all the things I used to do. And I understand that this change has been very hard on you, too. I want you to tell me about your feelings so we work this out together." This kind of simple statement can open up doors of understanding and acceptance that have long been closed.

Avoid Talking About Physical Symptoms

It would be nice if caring family members could listen to your complaints of physical symptoms and come up with a way to "fix" you. Unfortunately, that is not going to happen. Only the person with lupus can take the responsibility for living well. For this reason, Cowan encourages family members to avoid talking about physical symptoms. She feels it's best if family members don't start every conversation with, "How are you feeling?" "This is a futile discussion because no one will ever really know how another person feels physically," says Cowan. "We cannot measure our pain. We cannot take the pain out of the body and hold it in our hand and say 'You really want to know how much I'm hurting? Here it is; this is how much I hurt.' Pain is invisible, so people in relationships with those who have chronic pain have to believe that the pain is real, but they shouldn't continually remind them and keep them in that 'disabled patient' type of role where they're not in control."

The person with lupus also needs to learn a new way of communicating that does not focus on lupus. There is a natural inclination to want to make your loved ones understand how you feel. You want to say, "I feel awful; you just don't understand and so I'm going to keep describing how I feel until you get it." Cowan says, however, that "No one will ever understand how you really feel, so it's a waste of time to keep telling everyone around you the details of the pain and fatigue that plague you. It is impossible to feel another person's pain, so don't get hung up trying to explain it. Even if you cut your finger and someone else cuts his finger in the same spot, you will still experience the pain in different ways."

Talking about your pain is also counterproductive because if you have to keep explaining how you feel, you are forced to keep thinking about it. "The more you think about the pain," says Cowan, "the more you suffer. You're going to suffer less if you can redirect your thoughts off of the pain and onto something you have more control over. That doesn't mean your pain is going to miraculously go away; it means you won't suffer as much. The goal is to learn how to keep pain from becoming the focus of your life. This is the hardest hump to get over and accept."

Saying that you should avoid talking about your physical symptoms is not recommending that you enter a state of denial—just the opposite. Remember, you should start with a conversation that asks everyone in your family to acknowledge and validate your physical condition. Once you all agree that you are living with a very difficult circumstance, there is no reason to keep going over and over that.

> *Saying that you should avoid talking about your physical symptoms is not recommending that you enter a state of denial—just the opposite.*

Develop a Family System of Communication

Once family members acknowledge and validate that you have physical symptoms that are difficult to deal with, you can then begin to change the way you all communicate. Cowan recommends that you establish a neutral system that lets you communicate the way you feel at any given time without having to further justify, validate, or explain yourself. If your family wants to go ice-skating and you know that a trip out in the cold will make your already aching joints worse, you can simply say, "That's not something I can do today," without trying to make them understand all your reasons. Or, you can agree in advance that if you say, "This is a bad day," everyone will understand and accept your behavior without asking for an explanation.

There are many ways you can communicate without putting yourself in the patient role. Some members of the American Chronic Pain

Association use communication systems that are based on our understanding of traffic lights; this might be a green light day, or a red light day, or even a yellow light day of caution. Others draw little faces on the kitchen calendar with either a smile or a frown like the one in figure 7.1 to let everyone know nonverbally where things stand that day. And everyone in the family has this same right. If your spouse has had a tough day and just can't get the kids bathed at night, he has to have the right to say so. If your significant other just doesn't feel like doing all the cooking again, she should be allowed to call for some take-out without having to justify or explain.

> *Once family members acknowledge and validate that you have physical symptoms that are difficult to deal with, you can then begin to change the way you all communicate.*

General Communication Tips

The skill of communicating feelings and needs may take some time to develop, especially if your present method is either to shout or stop talking completely. The following communication tips, adapted from the *American Chronic Pain Association Family Manual*, will help you get started:

Avoid emotionally charged conversation. Recognize how you feel emotionally before becoming involved in a serious discussion. When

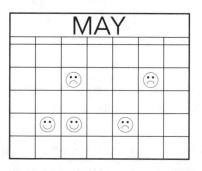

Figure 7.1—*A Family Calendar Can Let Everyone Know How You Are Feeling*

Your Basic Rights

- You have the right to say no.
- You have the right to do less than what is humanly possible.
- You have the right not to have to justify your behavior.
- You have the right to be treated with dignity and respect.

—PENNEY COWAN, EXECUTIVE DIRECTOR, AMERICAN CHRONIC PAIN ASSOCIATION

you or your listeners are emotionally upset, it may be difficult to concentrate or be objective. Sometimes timing is everything.

Make sure you are not in too much pain to concentrate or be objective. When discussing an issue that is important to a family member, everyone needs to pay attention. Pain can decrease the ability to process what is being said. You may agree to what is being said at the time, but when your pain is under control, totally forget the conversation ever took place.

Take responsibility for what you say. Whenever possible, try to speak in the first person. Avoid statements like, "We all know . . ." or "So and so told me . . ." Your emotions and feelings are yours: Say, "I feel . . ." If you are sharing a thought, say, "I think that . . ." And, if you are making a request, say, "I want . . ." It is not appropriate to believe that someone else can infer what you feel, so it's important that you express your own feelings and ideas. And remember that your honest feelings are valid—you have a right to them.

Listen to the feedback others give you. Three people in the room are all listening to the same discussion. If they were asked what they heard, it would not be unusual to hear three totally different accounts.

When people listen, they listen with their ears, their experiences, and their emotions. To ensure that a message is understood, ask others to state their understanding of what was said. This gives you the opportunity to clarify any misinterpretations immediately and keep the lines of communication open.

Don't beat around the bush; be direct about your needs. There is a lot to be said for getting directly to the point. If you need something, simply ask.

Don't allow others to tell you how you feel. Our feelings are unique. Unless we tell others how we feel, they have no way of knowing. If someone tells you how you feel, you have the right to state, in your own words, how you really feel. To ensure that people know how you feel, use statements that start with phrases such as "I feel . . ." or "I think . . ."

Remember that you have no control over other people. In spite of how well you communicate, in the end, you have no control over what others say, do, or think. Communication is only the beginning of action. To achieve the desired results, families must work together, respecting each other's points of view.

Finding Strength in the Family

Kim, now 24, was 17 when she was diagnosed with lupus. Her family has been her backbone of strength ever since. "My mom never let me get really down about this. Right away, she pushed me to find ways to deal with lupus. She always supported me and made me feel that everything was going to be okay. We joke a lot because humor makes all things easier to bear. And when I couldn't eat salt, fat, or sugar because of the medication I was on, my mom jumped right in to find new ways of cooking things. We'd go to the store together and then try new recipes; some of them ended up in the garbage, but it was an adventure rather than a disaster for us.

Communication Tools to Help You Express Yourself

- Be relaxed in the way you move, stand, or sit. Positive body language reflects self-confidence.

- Personalize. Use "I" statements to take responsibility for what you are saying.

- Be direct and clear. Get right to the point and state exactly what you want.

- Recognize the circumstances of the individual of whom you are making a request.

- Be willing to compromise.

- Know that you will not always get everything you want.

Penney Cowan, American Chronic Pain Association Family Manual *(1998). Used with permission.*

"Having lupus can be very scary and very lonely if you have to go through it by yourself. There were times when I couldn't go out with my friends because of my fatigue and I just couldn't do everything that they could do. This was really tough to face in high school. If I didn't have my mom to fall back on, I don't know how I could stand it. She was my friend at home who was always there. I think it's important to have someone like that—a friend, an aunt, a mom or dad, anyone—because it's hard to go through this without someone to pick you up when you're down or just to give you a shoulder to cry on. I know I need emotional support and, fortunately, I have it."

Of course it's nice to have family to lean on when you have a life-threatening illness, but some people with lupus are worried about being a burden to their families. For a while during her college years, Kim decided that she didn't need anybody and could live with lupus without her friends' help. "I decided that I was not different from anyone else. I decided I could go drinking, stay up late, and keep up with everyone else. I was determined and strong—I didn't need to lean on anybody. Of course, I wouldn't listen to my friends when they warned me that I was killing myself. But then one day, when I got really sick, I turned back to my family, admitted what I had done and asked again for their help. Now I know that I'm stronger when I can admit that I need someone to walk with me through this."

SEX AND LUPUS

What does lupus have to do with sex? If you're the person with lupus, you know! To begin with, you suffer extreme fatigue and when you hit the bed, sleep is your goal. You take medications that can interfere with your sex drive, and the body and joint pain make a roll in the hay more like a pounding over minefields. If that's not enough to kill sexual desire, if you are female and also have Sjögren's syndrome, you experience irritation and dryness due to lack of vaginal secretions. Some have skin rashes in delicate places and others have mouth or vaginal ulcers or sores that can interfere with sexual pleasure. None of this is good for your sex life.

The fact that you may experience sexual problems associated with lupus does not mean, however, that you have to add celibacy to the long list of lupus consequences. You can help improve your sex life in two ways:

1. Be vigilant and proactive about treating all the symptoms of lupus.

2. Address the psychological factors as well.

Adequate treatment of systemic lupus is the first step toward improving your sex life. Treatment with appropriate medications can increase your energy level, an immediate boost to your sex drive. Pain relievers can help joint pain, and there are lubricant creams that can relieve the irritation of a dry vagina. Antibacterial mouthwashes for mouth ulcers and steroid suppositories for vaginal ulcers are also very helpful if needed. You might also try to relax your painful muscles before sex with moist heat, warm baths, or compresses. Adding stretching to your daily exercise routine can help keep you limber and avoid the pain of physical movement. You might also experiment with different positions and with pillows or kneepads to put less of a strain on uncomfortable joints. Finally, if your sex life is dragging, talk to your doctor about the side effects of your medications. Some are known to decrease sexual desire.

The fact that you may experience sexual problems associated with lupus does not mean, however, that you have to add celibacy to the long list of lupus consequences.

If lupus lowers your libido, your partner may get angry or sad that you "no longer love me." Your partner's misunderstanding can lead to ongoing battles and hurt feelings all around. The psychological side of sexual relationships is built largely on the ability to talk about these feelings. To keep the relationship going, you have to talk about how the fatigue, pain, and complications of this disease affect your emotions, your sensuality, and your physical ability to have sexual intercourse. Remember, your partner can't feel your pain, cannot guess how certain positions hurt you, cannot know that your indifference to advances has nothing to do with your feelings for him—he can't know unless you tell him. You can soothe the psychological distress of sexual problems by communicating to your partner that you care. Your partner needs to know that you still find him attractive, even when you physically can't have sex. These messages make a world of difference in the way your partner will react to the adjustments he is being asked to make.

One more issue affecting your sex life, if you are female, is the use of contraceptives. When it comes to oral contraceptives that contain estrogen, you need to exercise extreme caution. In *The Lupus Book*, Dr. Daniel Wallace says, "Estrogen-containing contraceptives are not recommended for patients with SLE who have antiphospholipid antibodies, high blood pressure, migraine headaches, a history of abnormal blood clotting, or very high lipid (cholesterol or triglyceride) levels. These clinical subsets are associated with an increased risk of developing blood clots or having strokes." However, Dr. Wallace adds, "Progesterone-containing contraceptives such as Micronor do not have any specific lupus-related complications or concerns and are safe in SLE."[2]

> *When it comes to oral contraceptives that contain estrogen, you need to exercise extreme caution.*

Many doctors also feel that intrauterine devices (IUDs) should be used with caution because they are associated with an increased risk of pelvic infection, a dangerous consequence for someone with an autoimmune disease. Barrier methods of contraception such as diaphragms and condoms are perfectly safe. Spermicidal creams, sponges, and jellies are also safe.

If you should become pregnant, you'll find that living well with lupus during a pregnancy takes vigilant care.

PREGNANCY AND LUPUS

If you dig up an old medical book, you'll find that the standard medical advice to all women with lupus was not to get pregnant, and if they did, they should have a therapeutic abortion. Since 90 percent of the people with lupus are women and 90 percent of women who develop the disease do so during their reproductive years, this was devastating news. Fortunately, things have changed drastically for the better in recent years. Today, it is commonplace for most women with systemic lupus erythematosus to have happy, healthy babies—when they make sure that they and their babies are closely monitored throughout pregnancy.

Getting Pregnant

Timing is important for women with lupus who want to have a safe and healthy pregnancy and childbirth. Most doctors agree that it is best to plan a pregnancy after being in remission from lupus symptoms for 5 or 6 months. This gives your body the energy and health it needs to support the development of a new life.

Trying to become pregnant during a time of remission also makes conception more likely. During periods of active disease, you may have irregular menstruation or none at all; this, of course, makes conception difficult. Also, if you have significant kidney disease with your lupus, you know that dialysis is associated with minimal or no menstruation. And certain chemotherapy drugs that are prescribed during a flare interfere with ovulation. For all these reasons, it is wise to plan a pregnancy during a time of optimum health.

The Good News: A Low-Risk Pregnancy

Your chances of having a healthy, normal pregnancy and childbirth are the same as any other healthy woman in the general population if you meet certain criteria that put you in the low-risk category. These criteria include any one or more of the following:

> Today, it is commonplace for most women with systemic lupus erythematosus to have happy, healthy babies—when they make sure that they and their babies are closely monitored throughout pregnancy.

- Having discoid lupus or drug-induced lupus only

- Having mild SLE

- Having normal kidney function

- Having SLE that is in remission

- Being off all medication

- Having no sign of Ro (SSA) antibodies or anticardiolipin antibodies

If you meet these criteria, you can expect a normal pregnancy and childbirth, although you should have your pregnancy carefully monitored by both your primary care lupus physician and your obstetrician.

The Bad News: A High-Risk Pregnancy

There is a small group of women with SLE who are considered high risk during a pregnancy because certain health conditions indicate that the pregnancy may cause danger to the child or the mother. Given that a rare few of the women in this high-risk group will die due to lupus complications, a high-risk pregnancy is a serious matter that needs to be discussed at length with your doctor *before* conception.

The high-risk category generally includes women with any of these medical problems:

- Active lupus myocarditis (heart inflammation). The stress of pregnancy can lead to heart failure.

- Active lupus nephritis or reduced kidney function. If dialysis is necessary during preganancy, the risk of fetal death greatly increases.

- Severe and uncontrollable high blood pressure. Unmanageable hypertension can cause a stroke.

- Need for chemotherapy during pregnancy. Most chemotherapies (other than azathioprine) can cause fetal abnormalities and maternal infections.

Many women with these risk factors miscarry or develop serious complications that threaten their own or their babies' lives. For women who are at high risk, careful consultation with their physicians may result in a recommendation of adoption or one of various surrogate options.

The Middle Ground

In between the low- and high-risk woman are the majority of the women with lupus whose pregnancies might present certain problems, but who, with careful medical monitoring, can expect to carry and deliver healthy children.

If you find yourself in this middle ground, you should find an obstetrician who is thoroughly familiar with high-risk pregnancies (this doctor is called a perinatologist). The birth itself should be in a hospital where treatable complications can be easily managed. For this reason, home delivery or "natural" childbirth may not be possible. These are the kinds of issues you should talk over with your doctor long before your due date.

Flares

It is possible that your pregnancy can cause or contribute to a lupus flare, but generally the flare is mild and easily treated. Dr. Michael Lockshin says, "Women who conceive after 5 to 6 months of remission are less likely to experience prob-

> **Men with Lupus**
> SLE does not affect the male's sperm. Certain chemotherapeutic drugs can interfere with sperm production, however. Before beginning treatment with these drugs, some men choose to store healthy sperm for later use. Talk to your physician about this option.

lems with lupus than those who get pregnant while lupus is active. It also appears that having lupus nephritis before conception can increase the chance of experiencing a lupus flare during pregnancy."

According to Dr. Lockshin, the most common symptoms of these flares are arthritis, rashes, and fatigue. He also notes that approximately 33 percent of lupus patients will have a decrease in platelet count during pregnancy, and about 20 percent will have an increase in or new occurrence of protein in the urine. "But," cautions Dr. Lockshin, "it is important to distinguish the symptoms of lupus flare from the normal body changes that occur during pregnancy." For example, because the ligaments that hold the joints together normally soften in pregnancy, fluid may accumulate in the joints, especially in the knees, and cause swelling. Although this may suggest an increase in inflammation due to lupus, it may simply be the swelling that occurs during a normal pregnancy. Similarly, lupus rashes may appear to worsen during pregnancy, but this is usually due to an increased blood flow to the skin that is common in pregnancy. Many women also experience new hair growth during pregnancy, followed by a dramatic loss of hair after delivery. Although hair loss is certainly a symptom of active SLE, this again is most likely a result of the changes that occur during a normal pregnancy.[3]

Medications During Pregnancy

If You're Lucky

Some lucky women with lupus, approximately 6 to 15 percent, will actually experience an improvement in their symptoms during pregnancy.

All women are advised to avoid any unnecessary medications while pregnant. This is true for woman with lupus also, but some medications used to manage active lupus are absolutely necessary to continued good health. Your doctor will need to weigh carefully the risks and benefits of each medication.

According to Dr. Lockshin, most medications commonly prescribed for the treatment of lupus are safe to use during pregnancy, but always talk to your doctor before taking or discontinuing any medication during pregnancy. The following are what is commonly known about the effect of certain lupus drugs on a pregnancy:

- The steroids prednisone, prednisolone, and probably methylprednisolone (Medrol) do not get through the placenta and therefore will not harm the baby.

- Preliminary reports suggest that the immunosuppressive drug azathioprine (Imuran) and the antimalarial drug hydroxychloroquine (Plaquenil) do not harm babies.

- Low-dose aspirin is safe and is often used to protect against a complication of pregnancy known as toxemia.

- Dexamethasone (Decadron, Hexadrol) and betamethasone (Celestone) do pass through the placenta to the baby and should be used only when it is necessary to treat the baby as well. (For example, these medications might be used to help the baby's lungs mature more rapidly if the baby will be born prematurely.)

- The immunosuppressive medication cyclophosphamide (Cytoxan) is definitely harmful if taken during the first three months of pregnancy.

- Methotrexate and CellCept are harmful if taken during pregnancy.

Complications During Pregnancy

A pregnant woman with lupus should be closely monitored throughout the pregnancy by both her obstetrician and primary care lupus physician. Both will be careful to look for complications that might affect the health of either the mother or the child. Two situations to which they will be especially alert are the possible presence of antiphospholipid antibodies and complications due to kidney disease.

Antiphospholipid Antibodies and Miscarriage

"About 33 percent of lupus patients have antibodies that interfere with the function of the placenta," says Dr. Lockshin. "These antibodies are called antiphospholipid antibodies, the lupus anticoagulant, or anticardiolipin antibodies. These antibodies may cause blood clots, including blood clots in the placenta that prevent the placenta from growing and functioning normally. Since the placenta is the passageway for nourishment from the mother to the baby, the baby's growth slows."

This clotting usually occurs during the second trimester and Dr. Lockshin warns that pregnant women who have the antiphospholipid antibody may miscarry between the fourth and seventh month, or if the baby is large enough, may deliver prematurely. But the baby may be carried to term if preventive treatment is begun early in the pregnancy. "Most doctors," says Dr. Lockshin, "now treat pregnant women who have had prior unsuccessful pregnancies due to antiphospholipid antibodies with aspirin and heparin to prevent blood clotting in the placenta. Prednisone therapy does not help for antiphospholipid antibody complications, but should be used if lupus is active."

Kidney Disease and Toxemia

If you have severe kidney involvement with lupus, you may have a more difficult pregnancy than most women with lupus have. The most common problem is a complication called toxemia or pre-eclampsia. This condition causes blood pressure to rise, protein to be excreted in the urine, and fluid to collect in the legs and elsewhere. "If toxemia develops," says Dr. Lockshin, "the most effective treatment is to deliver the baby as soon as possible, even if the baby will be premature."

If you have kidney nephritis, you should talk to your nephrologist and obstetrician before becoming pregnant. If your blood pressure before pregnancy is high enough to need strong medications to keep it normal, or if the kidney function measured by creatinine clearance is more than 25 percent less than normal, a pregnancy would carry great risk for both you and your baby.[4]

Caring for the Baby

Caring for yourself during your pregnancy is very important for your continued good health, but it is also very important for the health of your baby. You'll be glad to know that there are no congenital abnormalities that occur only to babies of woman with lupus and no unusual frequency of mental retardation. Below, Dr. Lockshin answers the questions most commonly asked by women with lupus about their babies:

Will my baby be normal? The truth is that there are risks involved in having a baby when you have lupus, but it's also true that if you don't begin your pregnancy at an extremely high-risk level and you are closely monitored during your pregnancy, it is expected that your baby will be born healthy.

What are the risks to my baby? Premature birth is the greatest danger to the baby of a woman with lupus. This can happen when the mother has antiphospholipid antibodies, when she is very ill with active disease, or when she develops toxemia. However, the vast majority of premature newborns (especially those weighing more than 3 pounds 5 ounces) grow to be perfectly healthy. There is also a risk of miscarriage, primarily if the mother has the antiphospholipid antibodies.

Will my baby have lupus? If you are among the approximately one-third of the women with lupus who have anti-Ro/SSA and anti-La/SSB antibodies, your baby may develop a condition known as neonatal lupus. It's important to understand that this is not the same as systemic lupus erythematosus. It consists mostly of a rash (often brought on by sun exposure) and blood count abnormalities. Without any treatment, children with neonatal lupus generally have no trace of the disease by 3 to 6 months of age and it does not recur.

One rare complication of neonatal lupus, however, is more serious and is permanent. Some children develop a heartbeat abnormality, called a heart block, which results in a very slow heartbeat. The condition is treatable (sometimes an infant with this condition needs a pacemaker after birth), and the babies grow normally. But heart block is not a common complication. Fewer than 1 percent of all pregnant women with lupus, and fewer than 3 percent of all women with antibodies to both Ro/SSA and La/SSB antigens, deliver babies with this problem. Babies of mothers who have antibodies to neither or to only one of the antigens are not at all at risk for this heart problem.

Also, you'll be glad to know that these children who develop neonatal lupus are no more susceptible to developing adult lupus than are children who have not had neonatal lupus.

The likelihood that your child will develop SLE as an adult is slim. Most doctors believe the risk is about 1 percent—the same likelihood that your brothers, sisters, or parents will develop lupus.

Can I breastfeed? Many women with lupus have successfully breast-fed their babies. Some face difficulties if their babies are premature. In this case, you may need to pump your breast milk until the baby is strong enough to feed from the breast. You must also talk to your doctors about the medications you are taking to manage your lupus;

some may pass through the breast milk and be dangerous to your baby's health.

Growing Up with a Sick Mom

Sheri is one lucky lady. Despite lapses in her medical care during her pregnancy, today she has a wonderful 7-year-old daughter. "I had not yet been diagnosed with lupus when I became pregnant," Sheri remembers. "But because I had had previous miscarriages, the doctor ordered a lot of blood tests early in the pregnancy. He found that I had anticardiolipin antibodies and lupus anticoagulant antibodies, but never put it together that I might have lupus, and despite the previous miscarriages (which I now know are common in women with lupus who have these antibodies that cause clotting in the placenta), I received no further exploration into a diagnosis of lupus. The doctor did, however, prescribe one baby aspirin a day to prevent a blood clot or miscarriage." It worked! Sheri carried this baby full term (and even had total relief from her lupus symptoms during that time!). Her daughter Hope was born perfectly healthy.

It was another 3 years before Sheri was diagnosed with lupus. Throughout her young life, her daughter has had to adjust to having a mother with a chronic illness. "It hasn't been all bad," says Sheri. "In fact, it's given us some very special, and even funny, moments. A while ago I had severe, unrelenting chest pain and finally called the paramedics. As they were carrying me out the front door on a stretcher, I heard Hope in the background asking one of the police officers if he wanted to buy some Girl Scout cookies. To anyone else, this might sound like a coldhearted child, completely detached from her mother's suffering, but I just laughed because I knew better. Hope is used to living with a mother who has a chronic illness, and that's not a bad thing. She's had rides in the ambulance with me often enough to know that the paramedics, the police, and the doctors and nurses in the emergency room take great care of me.

"When I'm at home and not feeling well, we find ways to spend some wonderful time together. She'll write and illustrate stories and then read them to me. We spend a lot of time together in bed, reading to one another, watching movies, and doing manicures and pedicures. (I've found this is a good way to keep Hope still for a while when I can't take any more bouncing!) We play board games, too, with the coffee table up against the sofa and Hope seated on a footstool nearby. I delighted in teaching her Junior Scrabble and can't wait until she's ready to give me a run for my money in the grown-up version.

"When the weather is nice we move outside at the end of each day after the sun moves behind the trees (sun exposure is really bad for me). Outside, we'll play simple games like bubble blowing or ball bouncing. We also spend a lot of time in our hammock that's big enough for both of us. We'll snuggle together and discuss the shapes of the clouds and talk about how butterflies learn to fly. It's a wonderful time for us and it has taught me to savor these blessed moments we might not have found had it not been for my illness. We look for the silver linings in all the clouds that come our way, and usually we manage to find them.

Be Proactive

Living well with lupus means taking care of yourself, even when it's inconvenient and takes up your time. Margrey Thompson has taken a proactive approach to her life and it's paid off. "I have Raynaud's," says Margrey, "so I buy dozens of pairs of gloves and keep them all over the place. They're in every coat pocket, every pocketbook, in the car, and by the freezer. I take Plaquenil, so I see the eye doctor every 6 months to make sure it's not affecting my eyes. I have Sjögren's and the dry mouth can cause cavities, so I go to the dentist every 2 months. I get a yearly bone scan to check if the prednisone is causing bone damage. I'm not a hypochondriac. I'm taking care of myself and have received the benefit of a high-quality life."

"My beautiful daughter with the tender heart has learned a lot by having a mommy who's often sick. She has enormous empathy for others and a sweet willingness to help and comfort—despite her Girl Scout cookie pitch during my last crisis!"

LUPUS AND YOUR CAREER

Sometimes lupus has very little impact on a person's ability to work, but sometimes the joint pain, fatigue, or organ involvement forces a person out of a current job or out of work completely. When this happens, of course, the financial and social impact can be devastating. That's why most people try to keep working as long as possible.

To Tell or Not to Tell

Once you find out you have lupus, you may wonder, "Should I tell my coworkers and my boss?" The answer to that question depends on how your physical condition impacts your ability to function. If, for example, a flare is going to keep you out of work for long periods of time, or you need frequent kidney dialysis, or some days you just can't keep up, your supervisor or close coworkers need to know what's going on. Unless these people know you have lupus, they're likely to think you're lazy or slacking off or that you let other people do your work. Let them know what you have, how you're going to handle it, and how they can most effectively help you. Be direct and open with the people who need to know.

If you are able to continue performing your job responsibilities, you should not have to worry about being fired. Depending on your degree of symptom severity, the Americans with Disabilities Act (ADA) may help you retain or obtain employment if you think your job is in

> ### Resource Referral
> To obtain answers to general and technical questions about the Americans with Disabilities Act (ADA) and to order technical assistance materials, call (800) 514-0301. Or visit the Web site at www.usdoj.gov/crt/ada/adahom1.htm.

danger. The Civil Rights Division of the U.S. Department of Justice says that the ADA prohibits discrimination in all employment practices of individuals with physical or mental disabilities as long as the person meets legitimate skill, experience, education, or other requirements of an employment position and can perform the essential functions of the position. If your boss thinks lupus is cause for dismissal, be sure to contact the Department of Justice to verify your rights.

Finding the Right Balance

Being the boss can be a blessing as well as a curse when you have lupus. Gwendolyn Young, 45, president of Young Communications Group in Los Angeles, has experienced the good and bad of owning her own company while dealing with the flares of lupus. "I was diagnosed with lupus 14 years ago. One year after that diagnosis, I had a serious flare that put me in the hospital for 5 days with body systems threatening to shut down. That was when I decided that I needed to pay attention to what my body was telling me whether I liked it or not. Fortunately, now I have a mild case and most often I can run this very hectic and stressful business; I have 11 employees and we deal with major corporations in crisis and strategic communications. But at times like this week when I'm feeling exceptional stress, or when I don't follow basic good health practices with a positive mental attitude, I feel it. Before when I'd get that tired feeling, I would just push through and keep going. Then I'd have a flare with muscle spasms, joint pain, swelling, and hair loss. Now I know better. I tell myself that I need to stop, take time off, or work from home. I've learned to let some things go and not expect constant perfection. That's a significant mind and behavior shift for me. I continue to be driven, but I'm trying to balance my life now."

> *Before when I'd get that tired feeling, I would just push through and keep going. Now I know better. I tell myself that I need to stop, take time off, or work from home.*
>
> *—GWENDOLYN YOUNG*

This might seem easy for Gwendolyn to do because she's the boss, but at the same time, being in charge puts more stress on her. "It's difficult because on one hand I want to set a perfect example for my employees; I want to motivate them and keep them inspired to maintain the standards. But at the same time I know that I can't always live up to those standards. Although I don't want to make exceptions for myself, I've had to accept that I have to take care of myself if I want to keep working. This is a constant focus for me, but finding a balance that works is especially important for people who have lupus and want to have a career."

Changing Jobs

For a person with lupus, there are many circumstances that make it impossible to work. To name just a few: A long commute or a heavy travel schedule can cause stress that aggravates your symptoms; standing long hours can be unbearable on painful leg and ankle joints; long hours can exacerbate the exhaustion that makes any kind of personal or social life impossible and can cause continuous flares. Some jobs are just not compatible with lupus. But many people with lupus have found that there is a middle ground between working in misery and quitting. Here are a few changes some people have successfully implemented.

Ask for reassignment. Sometimes there are jobs within the same company that are more compatible with your health. Look into a lateral move.

Change jobs. Find one that is closer to home, less stressful, or requires less travel.

Switch to part-time work. If you can afford it, this option keeps you active and involved in life, but gives you time to take care of yourself as well.

Telecommute. Find a job that lets you join the millions of employees who now work from home.

Become an entrepreneur. Starting your own business that you can do from home allows you to set your own pace and work around your good and bad days.

When the financial, professional, and social benefits you gain from employment are important to you, it's well worth the time and effort required to find a way to stay employed and yet acknowledge that to live well with lupus you often have to make some adjustments.

"Lupus Has Changed My Life"

Deidre Paknad, 38, has founded two companies and is currently CEO of her second, R101. She has a nearly 20-year career in the high-tech world—she also has lupus. "I've had health problems since I was 20," says Deidre. "I've had bronchial inflammations, blue fingers and toes, skin rashes, and blood clots, but it took 17 years to get to a diagnosis that connected those events. Unfortunately, the initial blood clot was combined with dramatic fatigue and joint pains; a lengthy diagnostic process and little relief from the discomfort made it difficult for me to finish my first year of law school in 1984. I decided to take an extended leave from school to recoup, and ultimately decided on a career in technology instead of law." This experience was the first of many that would test Deidre's tenacity.

A decade later, Deidre founded her own company, CoVia Technologies, an Internet technology company providing infrastructure for business relationship networks for large corporations. It was so successful that Deidre and CoVia were inducted into the Smithsonian Institution's National Museum of American History for technology innovations in 1999 and again in 2000; the company and her personal profile are a permanent part of the museum's collection. "I loved what I was doing and was feeling very good about our accomplishments. I had built a wonderful place to work and had established some great business relationships with customers," says Deidre.

In summer of 2000, Deidre focused on raising the company's third round of venture financing of over $25 million. The process is a high-pressure one and required a great deal of travel. During that time, her brother was killed in a tragic accident, adding grief to her stress. "By late September, I was feeling awful. I was very tired, had recurring pain in my leg, and was getting concerned that maybe I was having a third blood clot. Then I began to feel all-over joint and muscle pains and fatigue. I couldn't get out of bed."

Deidre saw several specialists in an effort to diagnose what seemed like disconnected symptoms. Through a series of tests ordered by a hematologist and rheumatologist, she had the diagnosis of lupus by the first of October. "By the end of October," says Deidre, "I formally resigned from CoVia. I didn't have the kind of job that would allow me to take a leave of absence, but it was clear that I needed, at a minimum, a few months to recoup. The company needed leadership with constancy and I needed to deal with the idea that I now had a chronic disease that could kill me. This was a significant personal challenge for me, and I needed to give it my time and attention."

> *I needed to deal with the idea that I now had a chronic disease that could kill me. This was a significant personal challenge for me, and I needed to give it my time and attention.*
>
> —DEIDRE PAKNAD

At first Deidre contemplated retirement. "But I love being in business," she says. "I love doing deals and thinking about how to solve business challenges. I love being a person who uses resources to create positive change and who gets results. I'm not really a spectator, and it was distressing to think about becoming one. I started to think: If it is possible that my life could be cut short, how would I want to have lived it? What should be the lasting value of my life? And I was very concerned about how my young daughter would feel—and end up feeling much later—about this huge challenge and change in my life. I didn't want her to believe that hard work and effort might be in vain, and to be left with a sense of futility. I wanted her to know that when bad things happen, it is perhaps more important than at any other time to do your best."

Like most lupus patients, Deidre wanted information on lupus to help her understand her options. She first visited the Lupus Foundation of Northern California in San Jose. "Although this nonprofit organization had been operating in Silicon Valley for more than two decades," says Deidre, "they had fallen behind in using technology to help achieve their client-service goals. As soon as they offered to make photocopies for me, I realized how much I took for granted in the tech world and how little of that innovation and those solutions had reached our nonprofit community. In January 2001, shortly after her visit to the Lupus Foundation, Deidre founded R101, a nonprofit organization that helps other nonprofits acquire and implement technology. The Lupus Foundation was its first success story when its newly designed Web site and online library were unveiled.

"We go to the companies who have the software systems and explain that it would be to their benefit and the community's benefit to allow R101 to freely distribute those systems to nonprofit organizations. Most agree with us and give us the systems to distribute and even help implement the systems. About 20 companies to date have provided us with products, people, or capital to help us achieve this mission. I'm very happy with our success in the first 6 months. We've aggregated over $20 million in products and services and have already redeployed about $4 million of that into the community."

Today Deidre lives a very complete life and enjoys the same entrepreneurial challenges she did before her diagnosis. "I still work more than 40 hours a week, but this is different in two ways. First, I have reduced a huge amount of physical stress by reducing my travel; I traveled 100,000 miles for CoVia in the first 6 months of 2000. That amount of travel is debilitating to anyone, with the hauling, running, and urgency that goes with business travel. Reducing the amount of ground I need to cover to build a business from a global scale to just northern California allows me to retain energy. Second, and perhaps selfishly, I find it helpful to work with people whose circumstances are significantly worse than mine. It's humbling and it's inspiring. In a simple way, I have the opportunity on a daily basis to know that what I'm doing with my time is of lasting merit, and this creates a certain peace that is the antithesis of stress. Because I generally do experience symptoms on a daily basis, it also helps me keep my head above my physical discomfort.

> *Lupus changed my life, and it isn't a change that I welcomed. It has, however, brought me clarity which makes the living of my life richer and more meaningful.*
>
> —DEIDRE PAKNAD

"Sometimes people think my new entrepreneurial efforts are less ambitious or that my purpose is less serious now because I have lupus. It's really quite the contrary. I am as intent and intentional about building a great business as I've ever been. It's incredibly important to me that I get to do the kinds of business things I truly enjoy, and to leverage my experience; R101 allows me to do that without compromise. Lupus changed my life, and it isn't a change that I welcomed. It has, however, brought me clarity which makes the living of my life richer and more meaningful."

SOCIAL SECURITY DISABILITY BENEFITS

No one involved in the treatment of lupus or committed to the support of people with lupus recommends going on long-term disability if it can be avoided. Work is too much a part of our lives and a part of our identity to just give it up. Work is not only where we make our money, but it is also where we have friends and social and business contacts. This is where a large part of our productive time is spent. Work, to many people, is a source of self-respect and self-esteem. It is also the place that keeps us too busy to focus all our attention on our disease.

For some people with lupus, however, there is no other choice. The pain and fatigue, and sometimes organ disease, are simply too intense—they cannot work a full-time job. This was the case for Orlando. He was diagnosed with lupus 12 years ago at the age of 37, when he was suffering from a lot of joint pain, especially in the knees, ankles, and hands. "I was a heavy equipment mechanic," says Orlando, "and I thought maybe this kind of work was tough on my joints. I asked the guys I worked with if they felt like I did, but they all said no. In fact, they used to call me Hop-Along because I walked with a limp. Finally, my wife convinced me to go to a doctor and he did some blood tests. When the doctor told me I had lupus, I was shocked. I had never even heard the word before. I started right away on prednisone and Plaquenil and went back to work hoping for the best."

Orlando had always been a very active man who was good at his job and he expected to continue this way. "But then," says Orlando, "it got difficult for me to do my work. It was a very physical job and my bosses were very demanding and asking more and more of me, but I just couldn't do it. I was always so tired and in so much pain, but they thought I was just lazy and slow."

Of course, this caused Orlando a lot of stress. "I wasn't getting the raises I should have and I was worried that I was going to be fired. During this time, I admit I was feeling sorry for myself and I did and said a lot of things I'm sorry about. I know I was full of fear, especially the fear of losing my family (I thought maybe my wife wouldn't want me like this)."

Soon Orlando's doctor recommended that he apply for disability, but he wasn't ready to stop working yet. "I worked the best I could for another 3 years and then I started looking for some kind of desk job, like in the service department, but I didn't have the experience for that. Then I had a bad lupus flare and I had to take time off. That's when I started to think that maybe my doctor was right and that I needed to accept that I just couldn't do the things I used to do." So Orlando began the process of applying for Social Security disability.

Following the guidelines he read in a book, Orlando gathered all his medical records and filled out the forms. His first application was denied and so he decided to get professional help. "A friend referred me to a paralegal who had helped his wife qualify for disability pay and he took my case because he felt strongly that I met all the requirements." But Orlando's second application was also rejected.

"I had heard," says Orlando, "that it's common to get rejected two or three times, so I just applied again. But this put a lot of pressure on my life, and if there was anyway I could have gone back to work, I would have. Work was my identity and I was feeling very useless. This whole process of being rejected made me feel like I was asking for a handout. But I had to keep reminding myself that I had worked for years and now had a legitimate disability."

Finally, Orlando's application was approved (about 2 years after his first application), and he was paid retroactively to the date of his first application. "I still don't have any medical insurance," says Orlando, "because I have to be on disability for 3 years before I can get that, so disability pay isn't a quick answer to financial problems, but you learn to wait and do the best you can."

> *The experience of having this illness has taught me a lot. I found out how strong I can be—and how strong I cannot be. It has forced me to evaluate my expectations of myself and of others.*
>
> —ORLANDO

Even though Orlando has lost his job and is now on disability, he says he feels fortunate. "The experience of having this illness has taught me a lot. I found out how strong I can be—and how strong I cannot be. It has forced me to evaluate my expectations of myself and of others and to be more patient. Although physically I always feel the pain of lupus, I have learned to cope and accept my limitations. I try to be a good father, a good husband, and a good citizen, and I've learned to relax more and take care of myself. I've come to realize how precious life is—even when suffering is a part of that life. Now, I've accepted that this is my reality."

Filing for Disability Benefits

As Orlando discovered, Social Security disability (SSD) benefits can be difficult to get if you are not visibly disabled (paralyzed or blind, for example). If you decide that you cannot work and need SSD support, you will have to go through a lengthy and tedious process of applications, hearings, and appeals. You will most likely have to hire an attorney, and you will wait many months, if not years, for a final ruling.

Alec G. Sohmer, Esq., a lawyer from Brockton, Massachusetts, has built his practice on supporting the legal needs of people with disabilities. He knows the application process can be long and difficult, but he also thinks that with the proper legal help, those who are truly disabled by this chronic illness will eventually receive the disability payments they deserve.

"The first step in determining your eligibility," advises Sohmer, "is to complete and file a written application at your local Social Security Office. As considerable information is required to complete this form, you should visit or call the office beforehand to determine what supporting documentation is required.

"Because lupus is not listed as a disabling condition on the list approved by the Social Security Office, expect a claim rejection. The listed impairments are specifically described physical or mental conditions that are so severe that the Social Security Administration has determined that persons suffering from those impairments are considered disabled. If your claim is rejected, you should appeal because benefits will be awarded if it is found that your condition causes substantially the same degree of functional limitations as other conditions on the approved list.

"After receiving the initial rejection, you must then file for reconsideration. The request for reconsideration is the first step in the appellate process, which is also completed by application. (It is helpful to retain a copy of the initial application because the Request for Reconsideration application seeks substantially the same information. This will reduce the time necessary to complete the second application.) You should prepare a detailed list of each and every physician who has treated you. The list should include the physicians' names, addresses, telephone numbers, approximate dates of treatment, and probable diagnoses. As much as possible, you should include every physician who has seen you, whether or not it was specifically for lupus.

"If the reconsideration is denied, you must then file for administrative appeal. This step is where most lupus claimants are successful. The administrative judge must determine whether your condition causes the same degree of functional limitations as those listed. In determining what is a severe impairment, the administrative judge will consider any condition which significantly limits a claimant's ability to do basic work activities such as walking, standing, lifting, bending, understanding, remembering, using judgment, etc. If the case history is properly presented, you are likely to succeed at this stage. Unfortunately, the entire process can take 2 years from start to finish." (See figure 7.2 for the three levels of the application and appeal process.)

Although the process can be a long one, Sohmer offers these tips to reduce the delay:

1. Get started now.

2. Prepare a list of each and every physician seen. This list should include names, phone numbers, addresses, approximate dates of treatment, and probable diagnoses. Remember to include all physicians, whether or not your consultation with them was related to lupus.

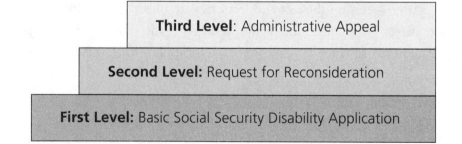

Third Level: Administrative Appeal

Second Level: Request for Reconsideration

First Level: Basic Social Security Disability Application

Figure 7.2—*Social Security Disability Application and Appeal Process*

3. Keep documents of medical records and how the condition affects your functional capacity on a daily basis.

4. Talk to an experienced attorney who understands both the condition and Social Security laws.

"Hopefully," says Sohmer, "your lupus won't be so debilitating that you will need to seek recompense, but in the event that it is, you should persist until you get the benefits to which you are legally entitled." You can locate more information about disability on Sohmer's Web site at: www.disabilityassistance.com.

REACH OUT FOR SUPPORT

Support groups can be an invaluable source of encouragement, information, and, of course, support that provides a better foundation on which to build all your other relationships. Even when family and friends are patient and encouraging, support groups can provide that understanding nod that a person who does not have lupus could never offer. No matter how supportive your family may be, only someone who has lupus can reassure you with the words, "I know just what you mean." It's one thing, for example, to hear from a professional that you need to exercise or that you should take your medications despite the side effects, but it's another thing to hear from someone who also has lupus how she's struggling like you to implement this advice. It's fine for a counselor to say, "You have to learn how to stop negative thoughts," but it's additionally helpful to hear firsthand stories about how someone in your same situation has tried that.

Resource Referral

If you need a lawyer in your area to represent you in a disability claim, you might begin your search with a call to an organization called **National Organization for Social Security Claimant Representatives (NOSSCR).** This is a group of lawyers who do nothing but SSD claims for any condition. (Fees are generally collected if they win the case). Contact them at (800) 431-2804.

Support groups also offer a place for gathering information. Many discuss conventional and alternative treatments and trade experiences about what works and what doesn't. Some focus on learning and implementing new coping skills, such as relaxation exercises, cognitive restructuring, and daily exercise. And almost all leave time for exchanging tips on diet, travel, family, work, and the like.

Even when family and friends are patient and encouraging, support groups can provide that understanding nod that a person who does not have lupus could never offer.

Knowing that you are not alone with your struggles can make life so much more bearable. Former Surgeon General C. Everett Koop has noted, "My years as a medical practitioner, as well as my own firsthand experience, has taught me how important self-help groups are in assisting their members in dealing with problems, stress, hardship, and pain. . . . Today, the benefits of mutual aid are experienced by millions of people who turn to others with a similar problem to attempt to deal with their isolation, powerlessness, alienation, and the awful feeling that nobody understands."[5]

Finding a Support Group

Support groups are out there, but you might have to look for them. Some are no more than a small group of people who meet occasionally to share a cup of coffee in someone's home; others are large, structured, and highly organized. It's a good idea to investigate a few (if available in your area) and pick one that you feel most comfortable with.

You can start your search by asking your doctor if he or she knows of any local support group. You can also call local or nearby city hospitals and ask if they know of or even sponsor such a group. The Hospital for Special Surgery in New York City, for example, supports a program called LupusLine. In operation since 1988, LupusLine is a national peer counseling and support program, providing ongoing telephone support by trained volunteers with lupus from home-to-home. The model has been replicated elsewhere in the United States and in British Columbia. A professional social worker initially screens calls and then "matches" the caller with a volunteer who has received extensive training in listening skills.

Charla de Lupus, a sister program of LupusLine, means "lupus chat" in Spanish. This is a bilingual peer health education program, available both over the phone, in person at New York City hospital sites, and through community outreach. Patients, family members, children, and teens are all welcome to use the program. This is the kind of support that's out there, if you're willing to do some digging.

You can also use the Internet to help you find the right support group for you. Edward Madara is the director of American Self-Help Clearinghouse, a problem-solving information bank listing over 1,000 national and international self-help organizations. At his Web site (www.selfhelpgroups .org), you will find information that will help you locate a lupus support group by checking for a possible local self-help group clearinghouse or contacting a national lupus group; or to start a group of your own. "Within a group," says Madara, "people pool their experiences, and members of the group see positive options that they may not have thought of before. I know how helpful this can be. When my wife was in medical school, she was diagnosed with lupus. I immediately called a lupus support group, and within the first 2 minutes, I felt a great deal of comfort hearing about the experiences of someone else who had this illness. Although this turned out to be a false diagnosis, I know firsthand from that scare how comforting it is when you realize that you're not alone."

Whether you're interested in finding an established group, forming a new group, or looking for an in-person group or an online

> **Resource Referral**
>
> To reach **LupusLine,** call (866) 375-1427 or (212) 606-1952 in New York City.
>
> To contact **Charla de Lupus,** call (212) 606-1952 between 9 A.M. and 5 P.M. (EST) to talk with the program coordinator, or call (212) 606-1958 for Spanish-language access.

group, Madara believes that essentially there are four characteristics of what he calls "mutual help" groups that make them what they are.

> *Within a group, people pool their experiences, and members of the group see positive options that they may not have thought of before.*
>
> —EDWARD MADARA

Mutual help. This is the primary dynamic process that takes place within the group; it is people helping one another and helping themselves in the process. Experiences are shared, knowledge is pooled, options are multiplied, hopes are reinforced, and efforts are joined as members strive to help one another.

Member-run. When members "own" a group, they provide a sense of belonging and reflect members' felt needs. If professionals are involved (and in many cases they are), they serve in ancillary supportive roles; that is, they are "on tap, not on top" as some groups describe it.

Composed of peers. Members share the same problem and experience, providing a powerful "you are not alone" sense of understanding, which can often lead to an almost instant sense of community at the first meeting.

Voluntary nonprofit organization. There should be no fees, and dues, if any, are minimal.

Do Support Groups Really Help?

The positive benefits gained from support groups are not at all subjective; they are a scientifically documented fact. Here are some examples of studies that have found a strong relationship between physical and mental good health and effective support groups:

- Results of a University of Chicago Medical School study of older men with diabetes found that those who learned self-care techniques and participated in member-run support groups were less depressed two years later, less stressed, had gained more knowledge, and rated the quality of their lives higher than those who didn't take such actions.[6]

- Similar research on group benefits has shown the value of groups for young diabetics, suggesting that "problem-solving groups can be more effective with young adolescents with IDDM [insulin-dependent diabetes mellitus] than conventional treatment."[7]

> **Resource Referral**
> You can contact the **American Self-Help Clearinghouse** by calling (973) 326-6789 or in New Jersey you can call (800) 367-6274.

- A study reported in the *Archives of General Psychiatry* in 1993 found that for persons at the early stages of skin cancer being part of a support group increased their chance of survival threefold over a 5-year period. Six months after the group sessions ended, two-thirds of the patients in the professionally assisted support groups showed an increase of 25 percent or more in what are called natural killer cells, which are cancer fighting cells in the immune system. No such increase was found in the control group.[8]

- In his noted research, Dr. David Spiegel of Stanford University found that women with breast cancer in a professionally run support group (where one of the professional facilitators had breast cancer) had a survival rate double that of the control group.[9]

- Adults with scoliosis who had undergone bracing or surgery and participated in a Scoliosis Association self-help group were compared to adults with similar treatment who did not participate in the group. Compared to nonparticipants, group participants reported: a more positive outlook on life, greater satisfaction with the medical care they received, reduced psychosomatic symptoms, an increased sense of mastery, increased self-esteem, and reduced feelings of shame and estrangement.[10]

Who can argue with results like these?

Avoiding Problem Support Groups

For all the good that a support group can offer, it's surprising how many people with lupus avoid them. Echoing the fear of many, 24-year-old May, who is a public accountant, says, "I don't know a soul who has lupus, so I was excited about attending a support group my doctor told me about. I sat among this group of about 12 women and prayed for some kind of encouragement because I was really depressed at that point. Boy, was I disappointed. Everyone griped and complained for 2 hours. It was like playing "Can you top this?" with horror stories. I went home and cried all night. That was such a discouraging and actually frightening experience that I never went back. I want to find a way to live well with this condition, and not spend so much time venting anger and frustration."

> ### Words to Remember
>
> It is one of the most beautiful compensations of this life that no man can seriously help another without helping himself.
>
> —CHARLES DUDLEY WARNER, AMERICAN ESSAYIST, EDITOR, AND NOVELIST, 1873

Kate Lorig, R.N., Dr.PH., an associate professor in the department of medicine at Stanford University and author of *The Arthritis and Lupus Helpbook*, understands why people like May avoid support groups. Lorig is presently involved in moderating and evaluating the effects of a 2-year-old online support group for 250 people with chronic back pain. She feels that there are three primary reasons some people have bad experiences with support groups.

Lack of a moderator. To be a positive, worthwhile effort, a support group has to have a good moderator who can keep the talk moving in a positive direction. Support groups without a strong leader can quickly turn into pity parties. Unless they are really well led, you sit and listen to one horror story after another as people play a game called my-disease-is-worse-than-your-disease. Good moderators are often health professionals such as a medical doctor, psychologist, or physical therapist, but not always. Many groups are led by laypeople who do an excellent job. Whoever is moderating has to keep the group from turning the meeting into a gripe session.

You may misunderstand the purpose of a support group. Some people find themselves involved with a very good group, but feel let down because they were hoping for more time to complain and share their misery. A good leader may say, "I understand that you all have had bad experiences, but I want to talk about what you are going to do this week to make things better." Well, that leaves no time for whining, does it? This is more of a challenge than an offer of sympathy, so when this happens, some participants who were expecting more handholding leave very discouraged.

The sponsoring organization may misunderstand the purpose of a support group. Sometimes "support groups" sponsored by health organizations are really more of a lecture program. They are called support groups because people do get to get together and talk a little bit, but the focus of the gathering is a lecture on a health-related issue. This too, can be very helpful—if that's what you want. But if you expect a give-and-take experience and end up in a lecture situation, you could easily get turned off to the idea of support groups completely.

To find a good support group, Lorig suggests that you contact a reputable organization and ask for a referral. You might try the Arthritis Foundation or the Lupus Foundation (see appendix for details). You might also ask your doctor if he or she knows of a local group or ask a representative from your health plan if they are sponsoring anything.

Looking for Support

Roxanne Black, 30, was diagnosed with lupus at the age of 15. "I had always been very healthy," she says, "but I started getting severe chest and back pain. At other times I'd have a rash from head to toe. This went on and on until I went into the hospital for a series of tests and finally found that I had lupus."

The high-dose steroid medications that Roxanne was given to treat the lupus made her hair fall out and her face swell up, and she was still in severe, constant pain. "That's just about the worst thing that could happen to a high school sophomore!" remembers Roxanne. "I was so upset and would always cry, 'Why me?' One day my mom told me that maybe I got sick for a reason; maybe I was chosen to make something good come out of this. And that made sense to me.

"I decided I wanted to start a support group for people with lupus in my area. I called the local paper and told them that I was 15 and that I had lupus and I wanted to find other people with this disease. The reporter agreed to do a short piece on my first support meeting and advertised that my lupus doctor would be the guest speaker. I was really nervous because I didn't know anyone with lupus and I didn't know if anyone else in my area had this disease. What if no one came? It was a risk, but about 30 people showed up and my lupus support group was formed.

"I ran this group all through high school. We had monthly meetings with guest speakers and then rap sessions in between where we would get together and talk. This became very rewarding for me and it eventually grew to have a mailing list of about 200 people, but still I hadn't found another teenager with lupus to talk to. Although we all had the same disease, we had different needs and interests. Many of the conversations were about the impact of lupus on a spouse and children and work, when I was wondering about how to deal with looking so swollen when the prom was coming up."

This problem helped Roxanne think more carefully about the fact that chronic illnesses affect people in different ways depending on many factors. She realized that someone with lupus whose primary symptom is joint pain can't really relate to someone with lupus with kidney failure. Someone who's 15 can't really relate to someone who's

40. That's when she came up with the idea to start another organization to connect people with any sort of disease or problem with others who were having the same experience.

"When I went to college," says Roxanne, "I started Friends' Health Connection. The idea was to connect people not only according to their diagnosis, but also according to their age, symptoms, work ramifications, hobbies, lifestyles, marital status, and so on. This way, people could custom-order a friend." To publicize the organization, Roxanne again wrote letters to the media. A reporter from *USA Today* picked up the story, then *CNN*, then *Time* magazine, and, finally, *Oprah*. "I was getting hundreds of letters from people all over the country and even from other countries. Now that the organization is established and successful, people have written back to me to tell me that the people they met through Friends' Health Connection have become their best friends, or have encouraged them to return to work, or to get married, or to have children. It's been so rewarding for me."

Since that time when Roxanne was looking for another teenager with lupus, her work has received much-deserved recognition. In addition to numerous state, local, academic, and service awards, she received the Daily Point of Light Award from President George Bush and became the spokesperson for the Youth Points of Light program. She received a medal from former United States Senator Bill Bradley and was honored with both the Sea Breeze Salutes Young America Award and the Jefferson Award for Service. She also has earned awards from the New Jersey Hospital Public Relations and Marketing Association, the Public Relations Society of America, and the National Speakers Association. Roxanne's story continues to be featured in media worldwide. "I would never have chosen to have lupus," says Roxanne, "but because I do, I have been able to touch many lives. These wonderful people who thank me for helping them have

> *These wonderful people who thank me for helping them have given me the answer to "why" I had to have this disease. My life has been enriched.*
>
> —ROXANNE BLACK

given me the answer to 'why' I had to have this disease. My life has been enriched."

Online Support Groups

At one time, support groups by their nature were gatherings of people with similar problems or illnesses. But today there are thousands of support groups whose members have never even met each other—they encourage and nurture each other online. Edward Madara tells us that there are four primary forms of online self-help support networks:

- Internet Web sites have interactive message boards and sometimes real-time chat rooms.

- E-mail discussion groups or listservs allow subscribing members to send and receive messages using e-mail.

- USENET news groups store messages on a computer in a central location, which can be read and answered by users.

- Dozens of various health or illness forums on the commercial computer networks like America Online, Prodigy, and Compuserve allow people to leave messages on message boards and meet with others in online groups, "chats," or conferences held at scheduled times.

Resource Referral

To contact **Friends' Health Connection,** call (800) 483-7436 or visit their Web site at www.friendshealth connection.org.

Whichever type you try, you'll find that online support has its pros and cons. On the plus side, as Madara says in his article, "Online Mutual Support Groups," "Online communication is an equalizer. In communicating with other people online, there are no visual distractions— no signs of social status, age, dress, weight, race, or appearance. People are seen for their words and ideas."[11] Also, some people prefer not to be face-to-face when they talk about personal and health issues. Online groups also serve many who would not be able to participate due to their location or disability. And most appealing is the fact that many groups are available 24 hours a day, 7 days a week.

On the minus side, however, online groups can have some drawbacks. Some people find them impersonal and miss the support of nonverbal communication like handshakes, hugs, and human presence. Also, if there are no ground rules and no moderator, you may quickly find that you've fallen in with a group of angry complainers. Anonymity gives some people courage to engage in serious verbal abuse or profanity towards others when they disagree. This is especially true online because here people will say things they would never say face-to-face.

When selecting online self-help groups for inclusion in his database, Madara looks for the following characteristics.

Is the group active and vibrant? This will be reflected by a fair number of timely, pertinent messages posted by a variety of people. The volume of recent interactive messages is one good indicator of an active group.

Are people helping one another? Look at the posted messages and see the degree to which people are sharing insights, successes, and information on helpful skills and resources. Exclude sites that reflect mostly "gripe session" messages that create a whining "pity-party" atmosphere.

Is the environment nonjudgmental and caring? Look for messages that make you feel safe and welcomed. Look for tolerance of differing opinions and feelings.

Is there an apparent sense of community? Because they have "been there," members should provide an understanding ear that no one else in the world can provide.

Is it nonproprietary? Exclude groups that have an explicit or hidden agenda of selling services or products.

> **Resource Referral**
>
> To begin your search for an online lupus support group, try these helpful sites:
>
> **American Self-Help Clearinghouse**
> www.selfhelpgroups.org
>
> **Dr. Koop's Community**
> www.drkoop.com
>
> **Support Path**
> www.supportpath.com

Is the group meeting people's needs? Similar to local community self-help groups, online groups have different values and personalities. Ultimately, a good group is one that best matches your needs and values.

A FULL LIFE IN SPITE OF LUPUS

As you think about how lupus affects your relationships at home, with your kids, at work, and with yourself, keep these words of Penney Cowan in mind: "I think people need to know that you can have a full life in spite of pain. When I first enrolled in a pain program for fibromyalgia 21 years ago, I really thought my life was at the very end. I went there with every intention of failing because I did not believe that anything in the world could ever help me. And I had absolutely no ability to help myself. I thought medicine was supposed to fix me. It never occurred to me that I had to be a part of my own treatment team.

"But that's where it's at," Cowan says. "The person with lupus has to be actively involved in living well, and we all have to accept responsibility for the quality of life we live."

CHAPTER 8

The Future

⚮

THE DIAGNOSIS OF lupus is no longer a death sentence. That
alone is progress. The advances made in treatment and diagnosis during the last decade have been greater than those made over the
past 100 years. That really is progress! In fact, although modern medicine has not yet found a cure for lupus and some people do die from
the disease, with current methods of therapy, deaths from lupus are
now uncommon. People with non-organ threatening disease can look
forward to a normal life span if they follow their doctors' instructions,
take their medications as prescribed, and know when to seek help for
drug side effects or new manifestations of their lupus.

Despite the rapid advances of recent years, however, there is still
no cure for lupus. Medical and scientific researchers around the world
are working to answer the many questions raised by this complex disease. They are striving to find the answers to questions such as:

- Who exactly gets lupus and why?
- Why are women more likely than men to have the disease?
- Why are there more cases of lupus in some racial and ethnic
  groups?
- What goes wrong in the immune system and why?

- How can we correct the way the immune system functions once something goes wrong?
- What treatment approaches will work best to lessen or cure symptoms of lupus?

Ongoing laboratory research, thousands of clinical trials, and government and organization-sponsored efforts around the world are seeking the answers to these and other questions. This chapter takes a look at how all this research offers hope for tomorrow.

GOVERNMENT AND ORGANIZATIONAL SUPPORT FOR A LUPUS CURE

The discovery of a cure for lupus will cost an immeasurable amount of time, money, expertise, determination, and persistence. Fortunately, there are organizations that are willing to commit these resources to a long-term battle against the disease. Collectively and individually, these groups are helping you every day by working to:

- Increase awareness of lupus.
- Provide education and information on symptoms, diagnosis, treatments, and management of care.
- Raise funds for continued medical research.
- Encourage more public and private partnerships and collaborative efforts to address this chronic illness.
- Encourage advocacy and support for lupus research.

Through their tireless efforts, you can hope for many more positive signs of progress in the near future. Among the many organizations particularly involved in lupus support (see the appendix for contact information) are the following.

United States Government. Congress enacted the Lupus Research & Care Amendment of 2000, which authorizes additional funds for lupus research and medical services. Congresswoman Carrie Meek (D-FL), who lost a sister to lupus, introduced this legislation in the House of Representatives. Congresswoman Meek has championed the lupus cause in Congress for nearly a decade. Senator Robert Bennett (R-UT) introduced the legislation in the Senate.

National Institute of Arthritis and Musculoskeletal and Skin Diseases (NIAMS). A component of the National Institutes of Health (NIH), NIAMS funds many individual researchers across the United States who are studying lupus. To help scientists gain new knowledge, NIAMS also has established specialized centers of research devoted specifically to lupus research. In addition, NIAMS is funding several lupus registries that will gather medical information as well as blood and tissue samples from patients and their relatives. This will give researchers across the country access to information and materials they can use to help identify genes that determine susceptibility to the disease.

American College of Rheumatology (ACR). A professional association of 4,000 American rheumatologists, ACR supports lupus research and disseminates the information to physicians and patients alike. Each year at ACR's annual scientific meeting, hundreds of papers on the latest research are presented. At the 47th Annual Meeting in 2001, there were 401 research papers presented on lupus. You can review abstracts of the latest studies on the ACR Web site (www .rheumatology.org) by clicking on "abstracts" and then using the search term "lupus."

Lupus Foundation of America (LFA). With over 100 chapters and subchapters and 80,000 people on their mailing list, this private organization publishes pamphlets and provides patient support and referrals. The foundation recently joined forces with the Department of Health and Human Services Office on Women's Health to host a 2-hour national town hall meeting. Leaders from government, health organizations, and the medical community connected with communities across the nation by satellite, making this meeting the largest-ever collaborative discussion of this life-changing and potentially fatal disease. This is certainly progress for a disease that few had heard of 10 years ago.

Alliance for Lupus Research. The Alliance is a joint undertaking by the Robert Wood Johnson family and the Arthritis Foundation. It was created in 2000 with a $12 million donation by Robert Wood Johnson IV to explore and focus on the gaps in lupus research, as well as on emerging scientific opportunities that will more quickly bring treatments to people with lupus. The Alliance is committed to an aggressive and targeted effort to find the prevention, treatment, and cure for lupus in the next 10 years. Using a strategic business approach, the Alliance awards substantial funding to research projects that will expedite improved treatments and lead ultimately to the prevention and cure of lupus. One hundred percent of all funds contributed to the Alliance go directly to peer-reviewed research opportunities. The Arthritis Foundation underwrites all administrative costs of the Alliance, freeing all funds raised by the Alliance to go straight into the hands of the lupus researchers. This arrangement allows The Alliance to make certain that scientists have the resources they need to allow lupus research to flourish and to accelerate discovery of cause, treatment, and cure.

Arthritis Foundation. The Arthritis Foundation is the nation's only voluntary health organization advocating on behalf of all people with arthritis and other autoimmune diseases including lupus.

WHERE WE ARE NOW

Research efforts have been successful in providing a general understanding of lupus and how it affects the body. Although there is still a lot to learn, we do know that lupus appears to be caused by a combination of genetic and environmental factors, and that disturbances of the immune system are responsible for the organ damage that is sometimes present. Let's take a summary look at these factors.

The Gene Factor

Studies in animal models of lupus as well as in families clearly show that lupus can be inherited, although the genes that pass on susceptibility have yet to be identified. Studies of twins have revealed that lupus is much more likely to affect both members of a pair of identical twins who share the same set of genes than two nonidentical twins or other siblings.

> *Identifying "lupus genes" will not supply all the answers. Only 60 to 80 percent of both twins develop lupus, pointing to the presence of other, nongenetic factors that contribute to the disease.*

The focus of many research studies is on the possibility of "lupus genes" that, if detected, could then be altered. This work is supported by the progress made in the Human Genome Project, which is identifying and cataloging every gene in the human body. This will enable researchers to tackle genetically complex diseases such as lupus and other autoimmune disorders.

Identifying these genes will not supply all the answers, however. Only 60 to 80 percent of both twins develop lupus, pointing to the presence of other, nongenetic factors that contribute to the disease, so research continues in other areas as well.

Environmental Factors

The environmental agents that may play a role in causing or worsening lupus are many and are under investigation. They include ultraviolet light, bacterial and viral infections, diet, various medications, and, perhaps, stress. The role of individual triggers, how they influence the course of lupus, and how the agents could be dealt with are all subjects of present research studies.

Immune Factor

Abnormalities in the immune system play a major role in lupus. Antibodies against multiple specific components of the nucleus are detected in most lupus patients, and are thought to be important in producing the inflammation and organ damage that occurs. It is important to recognize this root of lupus in order to categorize it as an autoimmune disease, but the precise reason for these abnormalities is unknown.

WHERE RESEARCH WILL TAKE US

There are many avenues of research being explored in the study of lupus to answer all the unanswered questions. Although is it impossible to review the thousands of studies focused on the cause, treatment, prevention, and cure for lupus, the following promising research will give you an idea of where we're headed.

Like most medical research studies, those examining the many aspects of lupus are divided into three levels of exploration:

1. Basic research

2. Translational research

3. Clinical research

Basic Research

Basic research is conducted in a laboratory and strives to understand lupus at a fundamental level and to develop or refine theories about the cause and treatment of the disease. This kind of research generally does not involve the use of human subjects. Studies of animal models of lupus are examples of promising basic research. Specific types of basic research include complement research, peptide vaccination research, and self-reactive B cell research.

Complement Research

David S. Pisetsky, M.D., Ph.D., and his colleagues at Duke University in North Carolina are studying the role of complement in the development of lupus. Complement is a series of proteins involved in the inflammation and tissue damage that occurs in people with lupus. Interestingly, people who are deficient in complement are at increased risk for the development of lupus. Dr. Pisetsky is conducting studies in a "complement-deficient" mouse to better understand the role of complement in the development of lupus and to determine whether administration of complement proteins might be a treatment for lupus.[1]

Peptide Vaccination Research

R. R. Singh and colleagues at the University of Cincinnati, Ohio, published a review of studies that aimed to discover antigens that activate the autoreactive Th cells thought to be involved in the development of autoantibodies. This paper reported that numerous laboratories are successfully using different approaches to find the sources of these activators. "With the successful identification of these putative autoantigenic epitopes," says Singh, "researchers now have the potential to develop peptide-specific vaccination as therapy for SLE. Indeed, vaccination of prenephritic lupus-susceptible mice with such peptides delays the development of autoantibodies and nephritis, and prolongs survival. Recent data suggest that peptide treatment can also influence established disease in older lupus mice. These studies offer new hope for a similar treatment approach in patients with SLE."[2]

Self-Reactive B Cell Research

Mike Carroll, M.D., senior investigator at the Center for Blood Research (a Harvard Medical School affiliate), is studying the effect of missing complement proteins on self-reactive B cells that make self-destructive antibodies. He says, "When certain self-reactive B cells come into contact with autoantigens, the B cells become deactivated and can no longer make self-reactive antibodies. In the absence of the complement system that helps transport these autoantigens out of the body, the self-reactive B cells fail to be deactivated, escape from the bone marrow, and circulate throughout the body, capable of producing large amounts of autoantibodies."

Translational Research

Translational research takes basic research one step further and involves the actual study of patients with lupus in the laboratory. Studies done on cells or serum from patients to better understand abnormalities of the immune system or on DNA to understand genetic associations are examples of translational research. Specific areas of investigation in this category are BlyS research and cellular waste disposal studies.

BlyS Research

William Stohl, M.D., Ph.D., of the University of Southern California, is involved in a promising translational research study. He is looking closely at BlyS (B lymphocyte stimulator). BlyS is a naturally occurring protein that stimulates cells of the immune system called B lymphocytes to produce antibodies. Previous research studies with animal models of lupus have found marked increases in the level of BlyS. Dr. Stohl is now studying the significance of BlyS in people with lupus to determine whether levels of BlyS correlate with disease activity and whether lupus patients' B cells are more sensitive to BlyS. If this study is able to demonstrate that BlyS is responsible for immune abnormalities in lupus, this would lead to the development of therapies to inhibit the production or block the action of BlyS to treat people with lupus.[3]

Cellular Waste Disposal Studies

Researchers suspect a genetic defect in a cellular process called apoptosis, or programmed cell death, in people with lupus. Apoptosis allows the body to safely get rid of damaged or potentially harmful cells. If there is a problem in the apoptosis process, harmful cells may stay around and do damage to the body's own tissues. Many research studies have focused on the hypothesis that the body's inability to clear up cell debris leads to SLE.[4] The following studies are just two of the many examining this theory:

- Cell biologists have confirmed that people with SLE tend to have low serum levels of DNaseI, an enzyme that degrades DNA and is responsible for clearing up cellular debris. The results of studies on DNaseI suggest that detection of high-risk cases may be possible through the analysis of DNaseI levels. Early diagnosis may also allow treatment with compounds containing DNaseI.[5]

- An English team led by Professor Mark Walport at Hammersmith Hospital is also looking closely at the link between cellular waste disposal and the development of SLE. This team studied both C1q (a protein in the complement system) and serum amyloid P component. Both are implicated in cellular waste disposal, and a lack of these molecules also seems to trigger the autoimmune response in SLE.[6]

> *Many research studies have focused on the hypothesis that the body's inability to clear up cell debris leads to SLE.*

Clinical Research

Clinical research involves studies of people themselves. New therapies are tested on people *only* after laboratory and animal studies show promising results. A clinical trial is a research study to answer specific questions about vaccines, new therapies, or new ways of using known treatments. Clinical trials (also called medical research and research studies) are used to determine whether new drugs or treatments are both safe and effective. According to John Yee, M.D., the chief medical officer at Veritas Medicine in Cambridge, Massachusetts, "Clinical trials are the only way to find out whether or not new treatments for lupus are effective and safe. Before any treatment goes to human clinical trials, it goes through a long period of study in the laboratory and then in animal models. Only those that are thought to have a high likelihood of having benefits for patients are entered into clinical trials. Of all the compounds that are examined as possible drugs, only approximately 1 in 5,000 will make it through the research process and be approved by the FDA for use in humans." Carefully conducted clinical trials are the fastest and safest way to determine treatments that work.

To demonstrate the value and power of clinical trials, Dr. Yee recalls the development of chemotherapy for leukemia. "The first chemotherapy for leukemia was given by Dr. Sidney Farber at Children's Hospital in Boston in 1947. At that time, leukemia was a uniformly fatal illness. Since that time, there have been many clinical trials for various chemotherapy regimens, so that now leukemia in children is curable in over 75 percent of cases. This has happened in a span of 50 years because of clinical trials that have organized the data on various treatments and their results. If it were just individual physicians trying different treatments, that information would not be collected, organized, and distributed to the medical community to be analyzed and understood. No treatment works 100 percent of the time, but clinical trials are an organized way to let us see what does work for many people, how it works, and how to make it better."

Clinical trials are designated as one of four levels of research. In the United States, the FDA requires these phases of research before it will grant formal approval for a product or treatment to go on the market for use in humans. The National Institutes of Health defines clinical trial levels as follows:

Phase I. Researchers test a new drug or treatment on a small group of people (20 to 80) for the first time to evaluate its safety, determine a safe dosage range, and identify side effects.

Who Sponsors Clinical Trials?

Clinical trials are sponsored by government agencies such as the National Institutes of Health (NIH), pharmaceutical companies, individual physician-investigators, health-care institutions such as health maintenance organizations (HMOs), and organizations that develop medical devices or equipment. Trials can take place in a variety of locations, such as hospitals, universities, doctors' offices, or community clinics.

Phase II. The study drug or treatment is given to a larger group of people (100 to 300) to see if it is effective and to further evaluate its safety.

Phase III. The study drug or treatment is given to large groups of people (1,000 to 3,000) to confirm its effectiveness, monitor side effects, compare it to commonly used treatments, and collect information that will allow the drug or treatment to be used safely.

Phase IV. Studies are conducted after the drug or treatment has been marketed. These studies continue testing the study drug or treatment to collect information about its effect in various populations and any side effects associated with long-term use.[7]

The following are particularly promising clinical trials associated with lupus.

LJP 394

La Jolla Pharmaceutical in California is a biotechnology company that is developing therapeutics for antibody-mediated autoimmune diseases such as lupus. The company is now conducting two Phase III trials for patients with lupus kidney disease (lupus nephritis) using the drug known as LJP 394. The trial is designed to arrest the production of disease-causing antibodies (specifically the antibodies targeting double-stranded DNA) without suppressing the healthy functions of the immune system.

According to Matthew Linnik, Ph.D., executive vice president of the company, "Our drug is designed to selectively knock out only the anti-DNA antibodies associated with the kidney component of lupus. This is a major improvement because all the other current therapies like steroids and cyclophosphamide wipe out the entire immune system and can cause major side effects. There are basically no known side effects with LJP 394. The compound is almost 97 percent DNA, so it is native to the body and the body handles it very well. And the results are impressive; in the last trial that we ran, the group that responded to the drug had one-third less flares than those in the placebo group. This drug is also an improvement because current therapies are used only after a person is in a flare and needs immediate treatment; LJP 394 is used to prevent flares. This should allow people to require far less steroids and cyclophosphamide. LJP 394 will have a huge impact on people with lupus-associated kidney disease." Dr. Linnik notes that LJP 394 is in its final Phase III trial. After review and approval it is hoped that the drug will be on the market in late 2003.

Stem Cell Transplantation

Stem cells are immature cells, which can differentiate into many types of cells and tissues. When stem cells are obtained from the circulating bloodstream, they are usually of bone marrow origin. Historically, after an individual has received a high dose of chemotherapy or radiation to kill malignant cells, stem cells are taken from the blood in order to re-populate an individual's bone marrow. This is called hematopoietic stem cell transplantation or HSCT. It is only in the last five years that we have seen the infusion of bone marrow-derived stem cells as an adjunct to chemotherapy treatment for lupus and other autoimmune diseases.

In the treatment of lupus, these transplants have generally been autologous, meaning patients are given their own harvested cells. (The transplants are termed "allogeneic" if the infused stem cells are harvested from a sibling.) If the aberrant, disease-mediating lymphocytes are largely destroyed by chemotherapy, it is hoped that the new stem cells will form a mature immune system without re-establishing disease. This means that they would form a normal immune diversity, similar to the immune system you had before the onset of lupus. In effect, stem cell transplantation is trying to turn back the clock on an error that occurred in immunity. This approach appears to be succeeding in the majority of patients treated with stem cell transplant so far.

In effect, stem cell transplantation is trying to turn back the clock on an error that occurred in immunity.

Ann Traynor, M.D., and her colleagues in stem cell transplantation at Northwestern University and Northwestern Memorial Hospital in

Chicago, Illinois, have studied the safety and efficacy of immune suppression and stem-cell infusion to treat SLE patients who experience persistent multiorgan dysfunction despite standard doses of intravenous cyclophosphamide. At a median of 3 years following transplant, 75 percent of patients remain without active lupus.[8] Says Dr. Traynor, "These patients improved continuously after transplantation, with no immune suppressive medication or with only small residual doses of prednisone. What was really surprising to us was the extent to which kidney, heart, lung, brain, and immune system continued to improve in the years following HSCT in most patients. Currently, stem cell transplant is being evaluated in a national, multi-institutional trial, comparing it to standard cyclophosphamide therapy." Dr. Traynor and her colleagues are now trying to understand why some individuals experience reactivation of lupus following HSCT, when most do not. They are also continuing to define the full potential of HSCT in lupus, in Crohn's disease, and in other autoimmune diseases.

BEING PART OF THE SOLUTION

One way to increase the likelihood that the future will be better for people with lupus is to participate in a clinical trial yourself. Many people

Advocate!

There are two special times to mark on your calendar: The Lupus Foundation of America has designated the entire month of October as National Lupus Awareness Month, and April 1 as National Lupus Alert Day. During these times, there is a major media push to increase awareness (and donations). Many local chapters organize volunteers to get out and distribute literature and take up collections. Call your local LFA branch and see if you can help!

just like you participate in clinical research for a variety of reasons. People who volunteer for phase II and phase III trials can gain access to promising drugs long before these compounds are approved for the marketplace. They typically get excellent care from the physicians during the course of the study. This care also may be free. Some people who are very sick or are not responding to standard treatments join clinical trials in order to receive new, investigational treatment. They are hoping that this treatment (possibly a new drug or a new combination of drugs) will work better for them than standard therapy. Other people participate in clinical trials to contribute to medical science and to help doctors and researchers find better ways to help others.

Finding Clinical Trials

If you choose to participate in a clinical trial, you will not be alone. At any given time, over 15,000 clinical trials in many areas of medicine take place in the United States, but it's estimated that only 5 percent of those eligible currently participate. Why? In the past it has been difficult to find these trials. Most people found out about clinical studies through their physicians or through advertisements in the newspaper or on the radio. But this was a rather random, hit-or-miss process that did not reach many eligible people.

Today, the Internet is changing the way people and trials are matched. The Web site Veritas Medicine (www.veritasmedicine.com), for example, is an online health resource focused on improving patient access to clinical trials and information about therapies in development for serious medical conditions. Veritas Medicine offers a comprehensive clinical trials database that allows people to be matched to clinical trials based on information submitted confidentially. The clinical trial matching tool is supplemented with information about current and investigational treatments developed by physicians from leading academic medical centers. Another site, CenterWatch Clinical Trials Listing Service (www.centerwatch.com), also offers a wealth of information related to clinical trials, such as a listing of more than 41,000

Benefits and Risks of Participating in a Clinical Trial

Before you sign up, you should know about both the bene-fits and the risks associated with clinical trials. The National Institutes of Health maps out some of the risks and benefits you should consider as follows (see the Web site www.clinical trials.gov).

Benefits

- Taking an active role in your own health care.
- Gaining access to new treatments that are not avail-able to the public.
- Obtaining expert medical care at leading health-care facilities during the trial.
- Helping others by contributing to medical research.

Risks

- There may be side effects or adverse reactions to med-ications or treatments.
- The treatment may not be effective for you.
- The protocol may require a lot of your time for trips to the study site, treatments, hospital stays, or complex dosage requirements.[9]

industry- and government-sponsored clinical trials, as well as new drug therapies recently approved by the FDA. Now it is easier than ever to be part of the solution.

Answers to Concerns About Clinical Trials

Participating in a clinical trial does not make you a guinea pig. The government has strict guidelines and safeguards to protect people who choose to participate. Every clinical trial in the United States must be approved and monitored by an institutional review board (IRB) to make sure the risks are as low as possible and are worth any potential benefits.

Beyond safety, some people have other concerns. They worry that if they participate in a clinical trial, they will be given the placebo (a

Questions to Ask About Clinical Trials

The National Institutes of Health is very involved in using clinical trials to advance the medical community's understanding of lupus. They also want the general public to be knowledgeable about how, why, and when clinical trials can be most personally beneficial. When exploring clinical trials, they suggest you ask the following questions.[10]

Questions About the Research

- Why is this research being done?
- What is the purpose of the study?
- Who is sponsoring the study?
- Who has reviewed and approved this study?
- Why does the research team think the treatment, drug, or medical device will work?

Questions About Your Participation in the Study

- Where is the study site?
- What kinds of therapies, procedures, and tests will I have during the trial?
- Will they hurt? If so, in what way and for how long?
- How will the tests in the study compare to tests I would have outside the study?
- How long will the study last?

"fake" treatment) rather than the tested medication that may help them. Dr. Yee understands this concern, but assures us that this is unlikely to happen in the case of lupus studies. "Placebos," he says, "are generally used to compare no treatment at all to the studied treatment. But when there is a standard method of treatment already in

- How often will I have to go to the study site?
- Who will provide my medical care after the study ends?
- Will I be able to take my regular medications during the trial?
- What medications, procedures, or treatments must I avoid while in the study?
- What are my responsibilities during the study?
- Will I have to be in the hospital during the study?
- Will the study researchers work with my doctor while I am in the study?
- Can anyone find out that I am participating in a study?
- Can I talk to other people in the study?
- Will I be able to find out the results of the trial?

Questions About Risks and Benefits
- How do the possible risks and benefits of the study compare with approved treatments for me?
- What are the possible immediate and long-term side effects?

Other Questions
- What other treatment options do I have?
- Will I have to pay anything to participate in the study?
- What are the charges likely to be?
- Is my insurance likely to cover those expenses?

use, as in the case of lupus, the trial will often compare the current treatment to the new treatment and no one receives a placebo." These trials determine if the new treatment is any better than what is already in use. That's why you can be part of a trial and be either part of the group that is monitored using the current standard of treatment or part of the group testing the new treatment therapy.

Some people stay away from clinical trials because they do not want to change physicians. But clinical trials do not replace your routine health care. In fact, Dr. Yee cautions that even though so much information is now available to laypeople, especially online, your own physician should always be your prime source of information. "It's important for patients to discuss with their physicians any decisions they may be making about participating in a clinical trial. The available Web sites are useful of course, but the information should be shared with the primary physician who will continue to stay involved with your care throughout a trial."

WHAT TOMORROW WILL BRING

Robert P. Kimberly, M.D., of the Division of Clinical Immunology and Rheumatology at the University of Alabama at Birmingham, has studied the research advances in the diagnosis and treatment of lupus. With high hopes, he predicts: "The next 25 years will contain remarkable progress in the understanding and management of SLE." According to Dr. Kimberly, we can expect to see the following:

- Specific genes that make one susceptible to SLE will be identified.
- Environmental triggers will be better understood.
- Assessment of individual genetic "portfolios" combined with advances in our understanding of environmental triggers will improve prevention efforts.
- New measurements of immune system activity will allow early therapeutic intervention.

- Biotechnology will provide more effective means of changing the activity of the immune system.

- The use of glucocorticoid steroids will decline and certain chemotherapy agents will no longer be part of the treatment regimen.

- Early, effective interventions will reduce lupus fatalities, which will be further reduced by aggressive management of the causes of these deaths.

There are many physicians and researchers who agree with the promising predictions of Dr. Kimberly. Dr. Daniel Wallace is one of them. These are some of the things he sees happening by the year 2015:

A national data network should reveal exactly how many lupus patients there are as well as their gender and their racial, ethnic, and occupational background. The gene or combination of genes that predispose one to SLE and the environmental factors (viruses, chemicals, drugs, etc.) that turn these genes on will be known. It should be possible to identify individuals at risk for developing the disease and perhaps to vaccinate them so as to prevent autoimmune reactions. By 2015, we will know why 90 percent of patients with lupus are women, and we'll be able to manipulate hormones to decrease the disease's severity.

Existing therapies for lupus will be fine-tuned and improved upon. An ideal NSAID that treats mild inflammation without any adverse reactions will be marketed. New-generation antimalarials and steroids that eliminate most of the side effects we associate with these agents should soon be available.

Down the line we will be able to fashion new immune environments that may eliminate lupus. Not only will people who carry lupus genes be vaccinated to prevent their activation, but also gene therapies, or placing messages into cells to produce or not produce proteins, will become important. Improved new ways of performing stem cell or bone marrow transplantation are theoretically capable of giving us an entirely new immune system programmed not to allow lupus to exist or become active. These are indeed exciting times for a lupologist![11]

Dr. Wallace's predictions are based on his intimate knowledge of where medical science stands now and where it is headed. These are not pipe dreams; they are possibilities that are already in the works. Medical researchers spend their days toiling to make these possibilities become realities. Of course, a universal long-term goal seeks to find the cause and cure for lupus, but researchers all over the world agree with Dr. Wallace that it will not be long at all before some lupus cases can be prevented, no one will die from it, and treatment will be both safe and effective.

This is very good news. But don't let these promises make you complacent in your own care. The hope of better treatment therapies for lupus is not an excuse to let your health care slide because "they'll be able to cure this soon anyway." While medical researchers are working so hard to find better ways to manage lupus, you must continue working hard yourself to follow doctor's orders to maintain control of the disease. That way, when new and better treatment therapies become available, you'll be in the best position to take advantage of them. Yes, you have good reason to hope that tomorrow will be better than today.

Appendix: Resources

Alliance for Lupus Research
1270 Avenue of the Americas,
   Suite 609
New York, NY 10020
Phone: (800) 867-1743
Web site: www.lupusresearch.org

American Academy of
Medical Acupuncture
4929 Wilshire Boulevard, Suite 428
Los Angeles, California 90010
Phone: (800) 521-2262
Web site: www.medical
   acupuncture.org

American Autoimmune Related
Diseases Association, Inc.
22100 Gratiot Avenue
East Detroit, MI 48021
Phone: (586) 776-3900
Web site: www.aarda.org

American Chiropractic
Association
1701 Clarendon Boulevard
Arlington, Virginia 22209

Phone: (800) 986-4636
Web site: www.amerchiro.org

American College of
Rheumatology
1800 Century Place, Suite 250
Atlanta, GA 30345
Phone: (404) 633-3777
Fax: (404) 633-1870
E-mail: acr@rheumatology.org
Web site: www.rheumatology.org

American Diabetes Association
1701 North Beauregard Street
Alexandria, VA 22311
Phone: (800) DIABETES
   (342-2383)
Web site: www.diabetes.org

American Massage
Therapy Association
820 Davis Street, Suite 100
Evanston, IL 60201
Phone: (847) 864-0123
Fax: (847) 864-1178
Web site: www.amtamassage.org

American Self-Help Clearinghouse
100 East Hanover Avenue, Suite 202
Cedar Knolls, NJ 07927-2020
Phone: (973) 326-6789
Fax: (973) 326-9467
E-mail: ashc@cybernex.net
Web site: http://selfhelpgroups.org

Arthritis Foundation
1330 West Peachtree Street
Atlanta, GA 30357
Phone: (800) 283-7800
Web site: www.arthritis.org

Association for Applied Psychophysiology and Biofeedback
10200 West 44th Avenue, Suite 304
Wheat Ridge, CO 80033
Phone: (303) 422-8436
Fax: (303) 422-8894
E-mail: AAPB@resourcenter.com
Web site: www.aapb.org

Friends' Health Connection
P. O. Box 114
New Brunswick, NJ 08903
Phone: (800) 483-7436
Fax: (732) 249-9897
E-mail: info@friendshealth
connection.org
Web site: www.friendshealth
connection.org

Lupus Acupuncture Network
8808 Harwood Avenue NE
Albuquerque, NM 87111
Phone: (505) 298-9550

Lupus Foundation of America Inc.
4 Research Place, Suite 180
Rockville, MD 20850
Phone: (800) 558-0121
Web site: www.lupus.org

Mary Kirkland Center for Lupus Research
Hospital for Special Surgery
535 East 70th Street
New York, NY 10021
Phone: (212) 606-1409
Web site: www.rheumatologyhss.org

National Center for Homeopathy
801 North Fairfax Street, Suite 306
Alexandria, VA 22314
Phone: (877) 624-0613
Fax: (703) 548-7792
Web site: www.homeopathic.org

National Certification Commission for Acupuncture and Oriental Medicine
11 Canal Center Plaza, Suite 300
Alexandria, VA 22314
Phone: (703) 548-9004
E-mail: info@nccaom.org
Web site: www.nccaom.org

National Institute of Arthritis, Musculoskeletal, and Skin Diseases (NIAMS)
National Institutes of Health
Building 31, Room 4005
Bethesda, MD 20892
Phone: (301) 496-8188 or
    (877) 22-NIAMS (226-4267)
E-mail: NIAMSInfo@mail.nih.gov
Web site: www.nih.gov/niams

National Kidney Foundation
30 East 33rd Street, Suite 1100
New York, NY 10016
Phone: (800) 622-901 or
    (212) 889-2210
Fax: (212) 689-9261
E-mail: info@kidney.org
Web site: www.kidney.org

**National Organization for
Social Security Claimant
Representatives (NOSSCR)**
6 Prospect Street
Midland Park, NJ 07432
Phone: (800) 431-2804
E-mail: nosscr@worldnet.att.net
Web site: www.nosscr.org

**National Osteoporosis
Foundation**
1150 17th Street NW, Suite 602
Washington, DC 20036
Phone: (800) 223-9994
Web site: www.nof.org

**Sjögren's Syndrome
Foundation**
366 North Broadway,
    Suite PH-W2
Jericho, NY 11753
Phone: (516) 933-6365 or
    (800) 475-6473
Fax: (516) 933-6368
E-mail: ssf@sjogrens.org
Web site: www.sjogrens.org

FURTHER READING

The Challenges of Lupus: Insights and Hope by Henrietta Aladjem (Garden City, New York: Avery Publishing Group, 1999).

Coping with Lupus: A Practical Guide to Alleviating the Challenges of Systemic Lupus Erythematosus by Robert H. Phillips (New York: Avery Penguin Putnam, 2001).

The Lupus Book: A Guide for Patients and Their Families by Daniel J. Wallace (New York: Oxford University Press, 2000).

Lupus: Everything You Need to Know by Robert G. Lahita and Robert H. Phillips, (New York: Avery Penguin Putnam, 1998).

Notes

Chapter 1

1. Lupus Foundation of America, "Introduction to Lupus," Lupus Foundation of America, 2000.
2. M. Lockshin, "Lupus: An Overview," In *The Challenges of Lupus*, H. Aladjem, ed., (Garden City, NY: Avery Publishing Group, 1999).
3. D. Wallace, *The Lupus Book*, (New York: Oxford University Press, 2000).
4. Ibid.
5. R.G. Lahita and R. Phillips, *Lupus: Everything You Need to Know*, (New York: Avery Penguin Putnam, 1998).
6. D. Wallace, *The Lupus Book*, (New York: Oxford University Press, 2000).
7. K. M. Holton, "Famous Lupies," Suite 101.com (www.suite101.com/article.cfm/4752/48630), October 1, 2000.
8. D. Wallace, *The Lupus Book*, (New York: Oxford University Press, 2000).
9. Ibid.; and W. J. Blotzer, "A History of Systemic Lupus Erythematosus," Lupus Foundation of America, (www.lupus.org.nz/history.html), 2000.
10. Lupus Foundation of America, "Introduction to Lupus," Lupus Foundation of America, 2000.
11. M. Stevens, "Joint and Muscle Pain in Lupus," Lupus Foundation of America, (www.lupus.org/topics/arthritis.html), 1995.
12. Lupus Foundation of America, "Introduction to Lupus," Lupus Foundation of America, 2000.
13. T. Provost, "Skin Disease in Lupus," Lupus Foundation of America, (www.lupus.org/topics/skin.html), 1995.
14. R. Schwartz, "Lupus and Fatigue," In *The Challenges of Lupus*, H. Aladjem, ed., (Garden City, NY: Avery Publishing Group, 1999).
15. D. Wallace, *The Lupus Book*, (New York: Oxford University Press, 2000).

16. R. Schwartz, "Blood Disorders in SLE," Lupus Foundation of America, (www.lupus.org/topics/blood.html), 1995.

17. J. Klippel, "Kidney Disease and Lupus," Lupus Foundation of America, (www.lupus.org/topics/kidney.html), 1995.

18. Ibid.

19. Ibid.

20. E. Chartash, "Cardiopulmonary Disease and Lupus," Lupus Foundation of America, (www.lupus.org/topics/cardi.html), 1995.

21. Ibid.

22. Ibid.

23. S. Blau, *Living with Lupus*, (Reading, MA: Addison Wesley, 1993).

24. E. Chartash, "Cardiopulmonary Disease and Lupus," Lupus Foundation of America (www.lupus.org/topics/cardi.html), 1995.

25. R.G. Lahita and R. Phillips, *Lupus: Everything You Need to Know*, (New York: Avery Penguin Putnam, 1998).

26. D. Wallace, "Systemic Lupus and the Nervous System," Lupus Foundation of America, (www.lupus.org/topics/nervous.html), 1995.

27. D. Wallace, *The Lupus Book*, (New York: Oxford University Press, 2000).

28. Ibid.

29. T. Provost, "Skin Disease in Lupus," Lupus Foundation of America, (www.lupus.org/topics/skin.html), 1995.

30. Ibid.

31. D. Wallace, *The Lupus Book*, (New York: Oxford University Press, 2000).

32. R. Zurier, "S.L.E. and Genetics," In *The Challenges of Lupus*, H. Aladjem, ed., (Garden City, NY: Avery Publishing Group, 1999).

33. D. Wallace, *The Lupus Book*, (New York: Oxford University Press, 2000).

34. Ibid.

35. R. Zurier, "S.L.E. and Genetics," In *The Challenges of Lupus*, H. Aladjem, ed., (Garden City, NY: Avery Publishing Group, 1999).

36. R.G. Lahita and R. Phillips, *Lupus: Everything You Need to Know*, (New York: Avery Penguin Putnam, 1998).

37. D. Wallace, *The Lupus Book*, (New York: Oxford University Press, 2000).

38. Lupus Foundation of America, "Introduction to Lupus," Lupus Foundation of America, 2000.

39. R.G. Lahita and R. Phillips, *Lupus: Everything You Need to Know*, (New York: Avery Penguin Putnam, 1998).

40. C. Welsh, "Black Women and Lupus," (http://lupus.about.com/health/lupus/library/weekly/aa021299.htm), n.d.

41. R. Lahita, "Hormones and Systemic Lupus Erythematosus," In *The Challenges of Lupus*, H. Aladjem, ed., (Garden City, NY: Avery Publishing Group, 1999).

42. D. Wallace, *The Lupus Book*, (New York: Oxford University Press, 2000).

43. Ibid.

44. R. Lahita, "Lupus in Men," Lupus Foundation of America, (www.lupus.org/topics/men.html), 1995.

45. M. Petri, "Lupus and the Elderly," In *The Challenges of Lupus*, H. Aladjem, ed., (Garden City, NY: Avery Publishing Group, 1999).

46. M. Rogers, "Lupus and Kids," In *The Challenges of Lupus*, H. Aladjem, ed., (Garden City, NY: Avery Publishing Group, 1999).

47. D. Wallace, *The Lupus Book*, (New York: Oxford University Press, 2000).

48. M. Rogers, "Lupus and Kids," In *The Challenges of Lupus*, H. Aladjem, ed., (Garden City, NY: Avery Publishing Group, 1999).

49. D. Wallace, *The Lupus Book*, (New York: Oxford University Press, 2000).

50. Ibid.

51. Lupus Foundation of America, "Introduction to Lupus," Lupus Foundation of America, 2000.

Chapter 2

1. M.C. Hochberg, "Updating the American College of Rheumatology Revised Criteria for the Classification of Systemic Lupus Erythematosus" [letter], *Arthritis and Rheumatism* 40 (1997): 1725.

2. R.G. Lahita and R. Phillips, *Lupus: Everything You Need to Know*, (New York: Avery Penguin Putnam, 1998).

3. M. Reichlin, "Laboratory Tests Used in the Diagnosis of Lupus," Lupus Foundation of America, (www.lupus.org/topics/laboratory.html), 1995.

4. D. Wallace, *The Lupus Book*, (New York: Oxford University Press, 2000).

5. Ibid.

6. C. Welsh, "Lupus and Sjögren's Syndrome," (http://lupus.about.com/health/lupus/library), April 12, 1999.

7. D. Wallace, *The Lupus Book*, (New York: Oxford University Press, 2000).

Chapter 3

1. J. Klippel, "Medications," Lupus Foundation of America, (www.lupus.org/topics/medication.html), 1994.

2. C. Aranow and A. Weinstein, "Nonsteroidal Anti-Inflammatory Drugs," Lupus Foundation of America, 1994, (www.lupus.org/topics/nserodial.html).

3. D. Wallace, *The Lupus Book*, (New York: Oxford University Press, 2000).

4. Ibid.; and O. Gluck, "Anti-Malarials in the Treatment of Lupus," Lupus Foundation of America,1994, (www.lupus.org/topics/malarials.html).

5. D. Wallace, *The Lupus Book*, (New York: Oxford University Press, 2000).

6. Ibid.

7. O. Gluck, "Anti-Malarials in the Treatment of Lupus," Lupus Foundation of America,1994, (www.lupus.org/topics/malarials.html).

8. Ibid.

9. R. Katz, "Steroids in the Treatment of Lupus," Lupus Foundation of America, 1994, (www.lupus.org/topics/steroids.html).

10. J. Klippel, "Medications," Lupus Foundation of America, 1994, (www.lupus.org/topics/medication.html).

11. D. Wallace, *The Lupus Book*, (New York: Oxford University Press, 2000).

12. R. Katz, "Imuran, Cytoxan and Related Drugs," Lupus Foundation of America, (www.lupus.org/topics/cytoxan.html), 1995.

13. Ibid.

14. D.T. Boumpas, H.A. Austin, et al., "Risk for Sustained Amenorrhea in Patients with Systemic Lupus Erythematosus Receiving Intermittent Pulse Cyclophosphamide Therapy," *Annals of Internal Medicine* 119 (1993): 366–9.

15. D. Wallace, *The Lupus Book*, (New York: Oxford Press, 2000).

16. R.G. Lahita, "Sex Hormones and Systemic Lupus Erythematosus," *Rheum Dis Clin North Am* 26 (November 2000): 951–68.

17. "R News: Health—DHEA for Lupus," CNN.com, (www.rnews.com/health/items/954371148.asp), February 2001.

18. Genelabs Technologies, "Drug Development Program: Aslera for Systemic Lupus Erythematosus," (www.genelabs.com/research/lupus.htm 2001).

19. M. Petri, "Treatment of Systemic Lupus Erythematosus: An Update," *American Family Physician* 57 (1998): 2753–60.

20. A.L. Drake, "Guidelines of Care for Cutaneous Lupus Erythematosus," *Journal of the American Academy of Dermatology* 34 (1996): 830–6.

21. Ibid.

22. S. Gupta, "Epidermal Grafting for Depigmentation due to Discoid Lupus Erythematosus," *Dermatology* 202(2001): 320–3.

23. J.F. Tremblay and W. Carey. "Atrophic Facial Scars Secondary to Discoid Lupus Erythematous: Treatment Using the Eribium:Yang Laser," *Dermatol Surg* 7 (July 27, 2001): 675–7.

Chapter 4

1. N. Flanigan-Ross, "Using Alternative Treatments," *webmd.com* (November 10, 1998).

2. C.D. Lytle, "An Overview of Acupuncture," Washington, DC: United States Department of Health and Human Services, Health Sciences Branch, Division of Life Sciences, Office of Science and Technology, Center for Devices and Radiological Health, Food and Drug Administration, 1993.

3. R.D. Culliton, "Current Utilization of Acupuncture by United States Patients," *National Institutes of Health Consensus Development Conference on Acupuncture, Program & Abstracts* (November 3, 1997).

4. L. Stone, "Lupus and Traditional Chinese Medicine," Acupuncture.com, (www.herbdoctor.com/Acup/lupus.html), n.d.

5. American Academy of Medical Acupuncture, *Frequently Asked Questions about Medical Acupuncture*, (www.medicalacupuncture.org/acu_info/faqs .html), n.d.

6. J. Horstman, "Acupuncture," *Arthritis Today* (May–June 2000): 78.

7. T. Monmaney and S. Roan, "Hope or Hype?" latimes.com, August 30, 1998.

8. J. Horstman, "Ayurvedic Herbs," Arthritis Foundation, (www.arthritis.org /ReadArthritisToday/1999_archives/1999_05_06explorations.asp), 1999.

9. A. Chopra, P. Lavin, B. Patwardhan, and D. Chitre. "Randomized Double Blind Trial of an Ayurvedic Plant Derived Formulation for Treatment of Rheumatoid Arthritis," *Journal of Rheumatology* 6 (June 27, 2000): 1365–72.

10. L.C. Mishra, B.B. Singh, and S. Dagenais, "Scientific Basis for the Therapeutic Use of *Withania Somnifera* (Ashwagandha): A Review," *Alternative Medical Review* 5 (August 2000): 334–46.

11. J. Horstman, "Ayurvedic Herbs," Arthritis Foundation, (www.arthritis.org /ReadArthritisToday/1999_archives/1999_05_06explorations .asp), 1999.

12. Ibid.

13. D. Wallace, *The Lupus Book*, (New York: Oxford University Press, 2000).

14. G. Wong, "Is Feverfew a Pharmacologic Agent?" *Canadian Medical Association Journal* (January 12, 1999): 160.

15. T.B. Klepser and M.E. Klepser, "Unsafe and Potentially Safe Herbal Therapies," *American Journal of Health-Syst Pharm* 56 (1999): 125–38.

16. "Potential Supplement-Drug Interactions," *The Arthritis Foundation's Guide to Alternative Therapies*, (www.arthritis.org/alttherapies/nature.asp), n.d.

17. J. Horstman, "Ayurvedic Herbs," Arthritis Foundation, (www.arthritis.org/ReadArthritisToday/1999_archives/1999_05_06explorations .asp), 1999.

18. "Herbs & Supplements: Fish Oil," The Natural Pharmacist, (www.tnp.com/substance), n.d.

19. A.J. Walton et al., "Dietary Fish Oil and the Severity of Symptoms in Patients with Systemic Lupus Erythematosus," *Annals of Rheumatoid Disorders* 7 (July 1991): 463–6.

20. W.F. Clark and A. Parbtani, "Omega-3 Fatty Acid Supplementation in Clinical and Experimental Lupus Nephritis," *American Journal of Kidney Disease* 5 (May 1994): 644–7.

21. W.F. Clark et al., "Flaxseed: A Potential Treatment for Lupus Nephritis," *Kidney Int* 48 (August 1995): 475–80.

22. L.J. Leventhal, E.G. Boyce, and R.B. Zurier, "Treatment of Rheumatoid Arthritis with Gammalinolenic Acid," *Ann Intern Med* 119 (1993): 867–73.

23. American Massage Therapy Association, "Massage Therapy: Enhancing Your Health with Therapeutic Massage," 1999, (www.amta.org).

24. National Institutes of Health, "Massage Therapy," in *Alternative Medicine: Expanding Medical Horizons. A Report to the National Institutes of Health on Alternative Medical Systems and Practices in the United States.* NIH Publication No. 94-006. (http://my.webmd.com/content/article/1680.51641), 1994.

25. Ibid.

26. American Massage Therapy Association, "Massage Therapy: Enhancing Your Health with Therapeutic Massage," (www.amta.org), 1999.

27. Ibid.

28. Ibid.

29. Natural Medicine Collective, *The Natural Way of Healing Chronic Pain*, (New York: Dell Publishing, 1995).

30. G. Hains and F. Hains, "A Combined Ischemic Compression and Spinal Manipulation in the Treatment of Fibromyalgia: A Preliminary Estimate of Dose and Efficacy," *Journal of Manipulative and Physiological Therapeutics* 23 (May 2000): 225.

31. National Center for Homeopathy, "Introduction to Homeopathy," (www .homeopathic.org), n.d.

32. J. Horstman, "Homeopathy," *Arthritis Today* (March–April 2000): 56–61.

33. J. Horstman, "Homeopathy," *Arthritis Today* (March–April 2000); Reprinted with permission.

34. "Magnet Therapy," The Natural Pharmacist, (www.tnp.com/therapy .asp?ID=1&Page=1), January 26, 2001.

35. B. J. Almond, "Magnet Therapy Reduces Pain in PostPolio Patients," *Texas Medical Center News* 19 (December 15, 1997): 8.

36. "Magnet Therapy," The Natural Pharmacist, (www.tnp.com/therapy .asp?ID=1&Page=1), January 26, 2001.

Chapter 5

1. A.C. Brown, "Lupus Erythematosus and Nutrition: A Review of the Literature," *J Ren Nutr* 10 (Oct. 2000): 170–83.

2. National Institute of Arthritis and Musculoskeletal and Skin Diseases, "Patient Information Sheet #9, Nutrition and Lupus," (www.nih.gov /niams/healthinfo/lupusguide/chppis9.htm), January 26, 1999.

3. Ibid.

4. B.H. Hahn and E.L. Mazzaferri, "Glucocorticoid-Induced Osteoporosis," *Hosp Pract* 30 (August 15, 1995): 45–9.

5. P. Sambrook et al., "Prevention of Corticosteroid Osteoporosis. A Comparison of Calcium, Calcitriol, and Calcitonin," *New England Journal of Medicine* 328 (June 17, 1993): 1747–52.

6. National Institute of Arthritis and Musculoskeletal and Skin Diseases, "Patient Information Sheet #9, Nutrition and Lupus," (www.nih.gov /niams/healthinfo/lupusguide/chppis9.htm), January 26, 1999.

7. Ibid.

8. P. Schur, "Some Thoughts Related to Lupus and Medications," In *The Challenges of Lupus*, H. Aladjem, ed., (Garden City, NY: Avery Publishing Group, 1999).

9. M. J. Rensch et al., "The Prevalence of Celiac Disease Autoantibodies in Patients with Systemic Lupus Erythematosus," *American Journal of Gastroenterology* 96 (April 2001): 1113–5.

10. R.G. Lahita and R. Phillips, *Lupus: Everything You Need to Know*, (New York: Avery Penguin Putnam, 1998).

11. N. Markle, "Aspartame, Diet Drink Poison," (www.bibleplus.org/health /ms_lupus.html), December 12, 1998.

12. C. Welsh, "Aspartame Internet Scare: Urban Legend or Medical Fact?" (http://lupus.about.com/health/lupus/library/weekly/aa011899.htm), November 18, 1999.

13. R. Dibner, *The Lupus Handbook for Women*, (New York: Fireside, 1994).

14. S. Epps, "Fit and Fabulous Despite Lupus," *Heart & Soul* 6 (November 1999): 60.

15. P. Schur, "Some Thoughts Related to Lupus and Medications," In *The Challenges of Lupus*, H. Aladjem, ed., (Garden City, NY: Avery Publishing Group, 1999).

16. National Institute of Arthritis and Musculoskeletal and Skin Diseases, "Questions and Answers About Arthritis and Exercise," (www.nih.gov /niams/healthinfo/arthexfs.htm), February 1997.

17. Ibid.

18. R. J. Shephard and P. N. Shek, "Autoimmune Disorders, Physical Activity, and Training, with Particular Reference to Rheumatoid Arthritis," *Exerc Immunol Rev* 3 (1997): 53–67.

19. "Osteoporosis: Self Care" (http://health.aol.thriveonline.oxygen.com /medical/osteo/seek.selfcare.html), October 2000.

20. R.H. Phillips, *Coping with Lupus*, (New York: Avery Penguin Putnam, 2001).

21. R.G. Lahita and R. Phillips, *Lupus: Everything You Need to Know*, (New York: Avery Penguin Putnam, 1998).

22. National Institute of Arthritis and Musculoskeletal and Skin Diseases, "Questions and Answers About Arthritis and Exercise," (www.nih.gov /niams/healthinfo/arthexfs.htm), February 1997.

Chapter 6

1. M. Castleman, "Depression in People with Chronic Illness," (www .depression.com/tools/health_library/coping/chronic.html), May 2000.

2. H. Shapiro, "Depression in Lupus," Lupus Foundation of America, (www.lupus.org/topics/depression.html), 1995.

3. National Institutes of Mental Health, "If You're Over 65 and Feeling Depressed," NIH publication no. 95-4033, (www.nimh.nih.gov/publicat /over65.cfm), 1995.

4. R.G. Lahita and R. Phillips, *Lupus: Everything You Need to Know*, (New York: Avery Penguin Putnam, 1998).

5. H. Shapiro, "Psychiatric Side Effects of Medicines Used in S.L.E.," In *The Challenges of Lupus*, H. Aladjem, ed., (Garden City, NY: Avery Publishing Group, 1999).

6. H. Shapiro, "Depression in Lupus," Lupus Foundation of America, (www .lupus.org/topics/depression.html), 1995.

7. K. Giuffre, *The Care and Feeding of the Brain*, (Franklin Lakes, NJ: Career Press, 1999).

8. Touch Research Institute, "Aromatherapy's Effect on Moods and Minds," *International Journal of Neuroscience* 96 (1998): 217–24.

9. M. Cameron and T. DiGeronimo, *Mother Nature's Guide to Vibrant Beauty and Health*, (Paramus, NJ: Prentice Hall, 1997).

10. Reprinted with permission of Prentice Hall/Learning Network Direct, a part of the Learning Network, from *Mother Nature's Guide to Vibrant Beauty and Health*, by Myra Cameron and Theresa DiGeronimo, copyright 1997.

11. Association for Applied Psychophyisiology and Biofeedback, "What is Biofeedback?" (www.aapb.org/public/articles/details.cfm?id=4), 2001.

12. Ibid.

Chapter 7

1. P. Cowan, *American Chronic Pain Association Family Manual*, American Chronic Pain Association, 1998.

2. D. Wallace, *The Lupus Book*, (New York: Oxford University Press, 2000).

3. M. Lockshin, "Pregnancy and Lupus," Lupus Foundation of America, (www.lupus.org/topics/pregnancy.html), 1994.

4. M. Lockshin, "Lupus and Pregnancy," In *The Challenges of Lupus*, H. Aladjem, ed., (Garden City, NY: Avery Publishing Group, 1999).

5. A. Katz (ed.), H. Hedrich, and C.E. Koop, *Self-Help: Concepts and Applications*, (Philadelphia, PA: Charles Press, 1992).

6. J. Gilden et al., "Diabetes Support Groups Improve Health of Older Diabetic Patients," *Journal of the American Geriatrics Society* 40 (January 1992): 147–50.

7. B. Anderson et al., "Effects of Peer-Group Intervention on Metabolic Control of Adolescents With IDDM," *Diabetes Care* 12 (March 1989): 179–83.

8. Self-Help Sourcebook—On Line, "Research Related to Self-Help Support Groups," (www.mentalhelp.net/selfhelp/research.htm), 2000.

9. D. Speigel, J.R. Bloom, H.C. Kraemer, and E. Gottheil, "Effect of Psychosocial Treatment on Survival of Patients with Metastatic Breast Cancer," *The Lancet* 8668 (1989): 888–91.

10. G.A. Hinrichsen, T.A. Revenson, et al., "Does Self-Help Help? An Empirical Investigation of Scoliosis Peer Support Groups," *Journal of Social Issues* 41 (1985): 65–87.

11. B. White and E. Madara, "Online Mutual Support Groups: Identifying and Tapping New I&R Resources," *I&R for a New Millennium* 22 (2000): 63–82.

Chapter 8

1. Alliance for Lupus Research, "Project Summaries," *Lupus Research*, n.d.

2. C. Henderson, "Results in Mice Suggest Peptide Vaccination Could Offer New Hope," *Vaccine Weekly* (November 1, 2000).

3. Alliance for Lupus Research, "Project Summaries," *Lupus Research*, n.d.

4. National Institutes of Health, "Systemic Lupus Erythematosus: Current Research," (www.nih.gov/niams/healthinfo/slehandout/research.html), February 2000.

5. A. Berger, "SLE is Caused by Cell Debris," *British Medical Journal* 320 (June 3, 2000): 1495.

6. Ibid.

7. National Institutes of Health, "What is a Clinical Trial?" (www.clinical trials.gov), n.d.

8. A. Traynor, "Treatment of Severe Systemic Lupus Erythematosus with High-Dose Chemotherapy and Haemopoietic Stem-Cell Transplantation," *JAMA* 284 (Oct. 18, 2000): 1904.

9. National Institutes of Health, "What is a Clinical Trial?" (www.clinical trials.gov), n.d.

10. Ibid.

11. D. Wallace, *The Lupus Book*, (New York: Oxford University Press, 2000).

Glossary

acupuncture   A form of holistic medicine that involves shallow insertion of fine needles into the skin at specific points on the body; can relieve pain symptoms.

adrenal glands   A pair of endocrine organs located above the kidneys; the outer layer (cortex) produces a variety of steroid hormones.

aerobic exercise   Exercise that requires cardiovascular endurance and that uses large muscles (primarily those in the legs) continuously as in running, walking, swimming, and cycling.

alopecia   Localized baldness.

alopecia totali   Hair loss all over the body.

anemia   A reduction in the number of red blood cells.

antibody   Serum protein made in response to an antigen.

anti-DNA antibody test   Blood test to determine if autoantibodies to deoxyribonucleic acid (DNA: the protein in the cell nuclei that makes up the body's genetic code) are present. The anti-DNA antibody is found in about half of those with systemic lupus and implies serious disease.

antigen   Protein that stimulates formation of antibodies.

antimalarials   Drugs used to prevent or relieve malaria.

antinuclear antibody test (ANA)   Blood test to determine if autoantibodies to the nucleus of the cell are present in the blood (also called the fluorescent antinuclear antibody test or FANA). The antibody is found in 96 percent of those with SLE.

antiphospholipid antibodies   Antibodies to a constituent of cell membranes seen in one-third of those with SLE (also detected as the lupus anticoagulant);

267

these antibodies can alter clotting and lead to strokes, blood clots, miscarriages, and low platelet counts.

anti-Sm antibody test Blood test to determine if autoantibodies to a particular protein known as "Smith" (found only in lupus) are present in the blood.

anti-SSA The antibody associated with Sjögren's syndrome, sun sensitivity, neonatal lupus, and congenital heart block (also known as the Ro antibody).

aromatherapy A healing treatment that utilizes the essential oils of both cultivated and wild plants that emit an aroma as they evaporate.

arthritis Inflammation of a joint.

atherosclerosis A condition in which fatty deposits build up on the inside of the arteries.

autoantibodies Antibodies that "attack" one's own tissues, causing inflammation, injury to tissues, and pain.

autoimmune Sensitive to one's self; the body makes antibodies against some of its own cells.

avascular necrosis of bone Death of bone caused by lack of circulation, which can be caused by steroid medications.

Ayurvedic medicine A holistic type of medicine focusing on establishing and maintaining a balance of "life energies."

basic research The first level of research conducted in a laboratory, which strives to understand diseases at a fundamental level and to develop or refine theories about the cause and treatment of the disease.

biofeedback A method of teaching people how to modify the body's response to stress by providing them with visual and/or auditory evidence concerning a body function, such as temperature, muscle tension, and heartbeat.

biopsy A diagnostic procedure that involves removing a small sliver of tissue, which is then examined under a microscope.

blood complement level test A blood test to determine the level of blood complement (a blood protein that destroys bacteria and also causes inflammation).

B lymphocyte or B cell A white blood cell that makes antibodies.

bolus therapy See *pulse therapy*.

butterfly rash A double-wing-shaped skin rash around the nose and cheeks; often seen in people with lupus.

cerebritis   Inflammation of the brain.

chiropractic   A system of therapy that holds that disease results from a lack of normal nerve function; it employs manipulation and specific adjustment of body structures (such as the spinal column).

chronic   Persisting over a long period of time.

clinical research   The highest level of medical research applied to human subjects.

CNS   Central nervous system.

CNS vasculitis   Inflammation of the blood vessels of the brain.

cognitive-behavioral therapy (CBT)   A type of psychological therapy that focuses on changing negative or non-coping thoughts and actions caused by persistent pain, repeated treatment failures, and the tendency of pain sufferers to focus their attention on their pain so intently that it comes to dominate their lives to the exclusion of other activities.

cognitive dysfunction   Causes feelings of confusion, fatigue, memory impairment, and difficulty expressing thoughts.

cognitive restructuring   Changing the way you think about your illness.

complement A group of proteins that, when activated, promote and are consumed during inflammation.

complementary and alternative medicine (CAM)   Health therapies that are not fully accepted by the conventional medical community.

corticosteroids   Steroids produced by the outer part (cortex) of the adrenal glands or synthetically produced, which are extremely effective in reducing inflammation and suppressing activity of the immune system.

cortisol   Hormone secreted by the cortex of the adrenal glands that is important for regulation and metabolism of fats, carbohydrates, sodium, potassium, and proteins.

CranioSacral Therapy (CST)   Involves gentle pressure and manipulation of the skull and spine and involves the fluid that flows around the brain and spinal cord.

Creatinine test   A blood test that measures kidney function.

cutaneous lupus   See *discoid lupus*.

DHEA   Dehydroepiandrosterone, a steroid hormone produced by the adrenal glands that helps produce the hormones testosterone and estrogen. A synthetic version called Aslera is awaiting FDA approval for the treatment of lupus.

discoid lupus   A chronic form of lupus (technically called discoid lupus erythematosus [DLE] or cutaneous lupus) that falls on the very mild end of the lupus spectrum as it affects only the skin.

DLE   See *discoid lupus.*

DNA   Deoxyribonucleic acid, a molecule responsible for the production of all the body's proteins and forming the body's genetic building blocks.

drug-induced lupus   Non-chronic, mild lupus that occurs after taking certain prescription drugs.

erythematous   Having a reddish hue.

estrogen   A female hormone produced by the ovaries.

flare   A sudden increase in symptoms.

gene   The basic unit of inherited information in our cells.

heart block   A rare but treatable complication of neonatal lupus that results in an abnormally slow heartbeat.

herb   A plant with a fleshy stem often used in seasoning or medications.

homeopathy   A system of medical treatment based on the use of small quantities of a substance that if taken in larger doses produces symptoms similar to the disease being treated.

hypnosis   A state of deep relaxation in which the subconscious mind is extraordinarily receptive to positive thoughts and suggestions.

immunity   The body's defense against foreign substances.

immunosuppressive drugs   Powerful drugs used to suppress a specific antibody; permits acceptance of a foreign substance, such as a transplant.

LE cell test   The first laboratory test ever devised (but infrequently used today) to diagnose lupus erythematosus.

lupus   A chronic inflammatory disease that can affect various parts of the body, especially the skin, joints, blood, and kidneys.

lupus nephritis   Lupus involving inflamed kidney tissue.

magnet therapy   The use of magnets placed directly over an area of pain to reduce the pain.

massage Manipulation of tissues (as by rubbing, stroking, kneading, or tapping) with the hand or an instrument for therapeutic purposes.

myocardium The muscle layer of the heart.

myositis Inflammation of the muscles.

neonatal lupus A non-chronic form of lupus usually limited to children of mothers who carry a specific autoantibody that crosses the placenta.

nephritis Inflammation of the kidney.

nonsteroidal anti-inflammatory drugs (NSAIDs) Drugs that reduce inflammation and pain but don't contain steroids.

NSAIDs See *nonsteroidal anti-inflammatory drugs.*

osteoporosis A condition in which the bones of the body become less dense and break easily; it can be a side effect of steroid medications.

pericardium The sac surrounding the heart.

perinatologist An obstetrician who specializes in high-risk pregnancies.

photosensitivity Sensitivity to light energy, especially the sun.

platelet A component of blood responsible for clotting.

placebo A placebo is an inactive pill, liquid, or powder that has no medicinal value.

pleurisy The chest pain that occurs when the lining of the lung (the pleura) becomes inflamed.

pleuritis An inflammation of the pleura (the membrane that covers the outside of the lung and the inside of the chest cavity).

pneumonitis Inflammation within the lung tissue, which may be caused by an infection or by lupus.

prednisone/prednisolone Synthetic steroids.

pre-eclampsia A condition that can cause a reduction in the amount of blood flow through the placenta, which slows down the delivery of vital nutrients to the fetus (also called toxemia). May be associated when severe kidney involvement in lupus is present.

protein A collection of amino acids. Antibodies are proteins.

pulse therapy (or bolus therapy) The administration of large amounts of corticosteroids intravenously over a short period of time.

range of motion exercises   Exercises that help maintain normal joint movement.

Raynaud's phenomenon   Spasms in the small blood vessels that restrict blood flow to the extremities and cause discoloration of the hands or feet (blue, white, or red) especially with cold temperatures.

remission   A disease-free period.

Ro antibody   See *anti-SSA*.

scleroderma   An autoimmune disease featuring rheumatoid-type inflammation, tight skin, and vascular problems.

Sjögren's syndrome   An autoimmune disease affecting glands such as the salivary and tear glands.

SLE   See *systemic lupus*.

steroids   Usually a shortened term for corticosteroids, which are anti-inflammatory hormones produced by the adrenal cortex or synthetically.

steroid-sparing drugs   A label indicating drugs (typically immunosuppressive drugs) that enable the dosage of prescribed steroids to be reduced without affecting the benefits.

subacute cutaneous lupus erythematosus   Lupus with characteristic skin lesions.

systemic   Pertaining to or affecting the body as a whole.

systemic lupus   A form of lupus (technically called systemic lupus erythematosus or SLE) that can affect almost any organ or system of the body.

systemic lupus erythematosus (SLE)   See *systemic lupus*.

thrombocytopenia   Low platelet count.

titer   Amount of a substance, such as antinuclear antibodies.

toxemia   See *pre-eclampsia*.

translational research   The second level of research that involves the study of actual patients in the laboratory.

UCTD   See *undifferentiated connective tissue disease*.

undifferentiated connective tissue disease (UCTD)   An illness similar to lupus that does not meet the diagnostic criteria for lupus set by the American College of Rheumatology. It is rarely organ threatening and less serious than SLE.

Index

A

Acupuncture
   description of, 103–106
   safety guidelines for, 106–108
Acupuncturists, 107, 108
Aerobic exercise, 148, 150, 152–153
African American women, 33
Age at onset, 34
Aladjem, Henrietta, 99
Alcohol, 85, 146
Alfalfa, 113
Alliance for Lupus Research, 236
Alopecia (hair loss)
   as lupus symptom, 11, 13, 14, 16, 26
   pregnancy and, 204
   steroids and, 77, 228
   treatment for, 72, 91–92, 96
Alopecia totalis, 26
American Chronic Pain Association
   (ACPA), 190, 193–194, 195
American College of Rheumatology
   (ACR), 4, 24, 45, 52–53, 109, 235
American Massage Therapy
   Association, 120, 121
American Self-Help Clearinghouse,
   225, 232
Americans with Disabilities Act (ADA),
   210–211
Anemia
   fatigue and, 17
   gastric bleeding and, 70

hemoglobin and hematocrit, 59
   iron supplements and, 139
   as lupus symptom, 11, 19, 40
Antibiotics, 29–30
Antibodies, defined, 5
Antibody tests, 60
Anticardiolipin (ACL) antibody test, 60
Anti-DNA antibody test, 55, 57
Antimalarial drugs
   description of, 71–73
   side effects of, 73–74, 161
   for skin problems, 93
Antinuclear antibody test (ANA), 41,
   42, 54, 55–57
Anti-Sm antibody test, 55, 58
Apoptosis, 240
Apresoline (hydralazinc), 3, 56
Aralen (chloroquine), 72, 73, 74
Aranow, Dr. Cynthia, 69
Aromatherapy, 178–181
Aromatic amines, 27
Arthritis. *See also* Rheumatoid arthritis
   homeopathy for, 125, 126
   lupus, 11, 12–14
   magnet therapy for, 126–128
   rheumatoid, 6, 14, 41, 60, 62, 63
   as symptom, 40, 53
Arthritis Foundation, 100, 114, 125,
   227, 236
Ashwagandha, 109–110
Aslera (prasterone), 88, 89

273

Aspartame, 33, 145–146

Aspirin
  blood clotting and, 70, 85
  defined, 69
  kidney problems and, 21
  pregnancy and, 204

Atabrine (quinacrine), 72, 73, 74

Autoantibodies
  defined, 5, 54–55
  research on, 239
  testing for, 55–58

Autoimmune diseases, 5, 6, 63

Avascular necrosis of bone, 78

Azathioprine (Imuran)
  description of, 80, 81, 82, 86
  pregnancy and, 202, 204
  skin problems and, 93

B

Babies. *See also* Pregnancy
  neonatal lupus, 4–5, 35–36, 207
  questions about, 206–208

Bennett, Robert, 235

Benson, Dr. Herbert, 178

Beta-carotene, 133

Betamethasone (Celestone), 204

Biofeedback, 182

Black, Roxanne, 227–230

Blood complement level test, 55, 58

Blood disorders/abnormalities,
    19–20, 54

Blood pressure, high (hypertension)
  cardiovascular disease and, 136
  corticosteroids and, 78
  NSAIDs and, 70
  pregnancy and, 202, 206
  salt intake and, 136, 139

BlyS research, 240

Bolus therapy, 76–77

Bradley, Bill, 229

Breast implants, 6–7, 8, 28

Breathing, deep, 174–175

Brown, Dr. Amy Christine, 132,
    134, 135

Bush, George, 229

Butterfly rash, 14–15, 53

C

Calcium, 79, 133, 140–141

Cameron, Myra, 178–179

Cardiopulmonary complications, 22–23

Cardiovascular disease, 136

Career issues
  changing jobs, 212–213
  Deidre Paknad's story, 213–216
  finding balance, 211–212
  telling boss/coworkers, 210–211

Carpenter, Virginia, 103

Carroll, Dr. Mike, 239

Cataracts, 78

Cause of lupus, 5, 236–238. *See also*
    Triggers

Cazanave, Pierre, 9

Celiac disease, 145

CellCept (mycophenolate mofetil),
    83, 205

Cellular waste disposal studies, 240–241

CenterWatch Clinical Trials Listing
    Service, 246

Charla de Lupus, 223

Chartash, Dr. Elliot, 22

Chemical factors, 27–28

Children
  babies, 206–208
  with lupus, 35–37
  of a sick mom, 208–210
  steroids and, 79

Chiropractic treatment, 121–123

Chlorambucil (Leukeran), 82

Cholesterol, high
  alcohol and, 146
  antimalarials and, 73
  lupus and, 23
  steroids and, 78, 79, 142

Clinical trials
  defined, 241
  levels of, 242–243
  LJP 394, 243–244

participation in, 245–250
sponsors of, 242
stem cell transplantation, 244–245
Clothing, sun-protected, 92
Clotting disturbances, 11, 19–20
CNS vasculitis, 24
Coagulation tests, 60
Cognitive dysfunction, 25, 110
Cognitive-behavioral therapy
  acceptance of lupus, 165–167
  defined, 164–165
  negative patterns, 167–169
  positive thinking, 170
  self-talk, 169
Complement research, 238–239
Complementary and alternative medicine (CAM)
  acupuncture, 103–108
  cautions regarding, 100–101
  chiropractic treatment, 121–123
  craniosacral therapy, 123
  herbs, 108–114
  homeopathy, 123–126
  magnet therapy, 126–128
  massage, 116–121
  nutritional supplements, 114–116, 139
  personal experimentation with, 129
  plotting progress, 101–103
Contraceptives, oral, 30, 199–200
Corticosteroids
  commonly used, 76
  defined, 75
  prednisone, 43, 75–76, 84, 85, 93,
   142, 204, 205, 209
  side effects of, 77–80
  for skin problems, 91–92, 93
Cortisone, 10, 75, 78, 80
Cowan, Penney, 190–193, 195, 232
Craniosacral therapy, 123
Cure for lupus
  organizations working toward,
   234–236
  participation in clinical trials and,
   245–250

predictions about, 250–252
research efforts, 236–245
Cutaneous lupus. *See also* Skin problems
  antimalarial drugs for, 72
  defined, 3, 90
  hair loss and, 26, 96
  lesions, 14, 95–96
Cyclophosphamide (Cytoxan)
  description of, 80–81
  for lupus nephritis, 81–82, 86, 87
  pregnancy and, 205
  for skin problems, 93

D

Dapsone, 93
Deep breathing, 174–175
Deltra. *See* Prednisone
Depression
  causes of, 160–162
  exercise for, 147
  lupus and, 157–158
  symptoms of, 158–159
  treatment of, 162–163
Dermatologists
  American Academy of Dermatology,
   90, 93, 94–95
  vs. rheumatologists, 96
Dexamethasone (Decadron, Hexadrol),
  76, 204
DHEA, 85, 88–90
Diabetes
  acupuncture and, 107
  as autoimmune disease, 6
  steroid-induced, 78, 142
  support groups, 224–225
Diagnosis
  criteria for, 52–54
  difficulty of, 41–42
  doctors and, 44–51
  illnesses with similar symptoms,
   62–64
  laboratory tests, 54–61
  second opinions, 51
  self-test, 40

Diagnosis, *continued*
   tale of misdiagnosis, 42–44
   three factors of, 61
   your role in, 39–41, 52
Diaphragm breathing, 174–175
Diet
   aspartame, 33, 145–146
   cardiovascular disease and, 136
   drug side effects and, 140–142
   food allergies, 145–146
   foods to avoid, 134–135
   foods to focus on, 132–134
   guidelines for eating well, 131–132
   hunger caused by steroids, 142–145
   Karen Kaufman's story, 136–140
   kidney disease and, 135–136
   nutritional supplements, 114–116, 139
   vegetarian, 134, 138
Disability benefits
   filing for, 218–221
   Orlando's story, 216–218
Discoid lupus erythematosus (DLE).
   See also Skin problems
   antimalarial drugs for, 72
   defined, 3, 90
   hair loss and, 26, 96
   lesions, 14, 95–96
DNA (Deoxyribonucleic acid), 57
Doctors
   diagnosis and, 44–51
   rheumatologists vs. dermatolo-
      gists, 96
Drug-induced lupus, 3, 29, 35
Drugs. *See* Medications for treatment

E

Echinacea, 113, 135
Erythrocyte sedimentation rate
   (ESR), 59
Estrogen, 30, 34, 89, 199
Exercise
   aerobic, 150, 152–153
   beginning program of, 147–148
   importance of, 146–147

   increasing level of, 147
   Margrey Thompson's story, 148–150
   range of motion, 150–151
   signs of too much, 154–155
   strength training, 150, 153–154
   stretching, 150, 151–152
   water exercise classes, 148

F

Family life
   communication system for, 193–194
   communication tips, 194–196
   communication tools, 197
   effects of lupus on, 189–192
   growing up with sick mom, 208–210
   strength and support from, 196–198
   talking about symptoms, 192–193
   your basic rights, 195
Famous people with lupus, 5, 36
Farber, Dr. Sidney, 242
Fat intake
   reasons to reduce, 134, 135
   tips for limiting, 143
Fatigue, 11, 12, 16–17
Fever, 17, 18
Feverfew, 110, 111–112
Fish oils, 114–115, 139
Flares
   defined, 18
   DHEA and, 89
   drugs that can trigger, 29–30
   exercise and, 146, 150, 155
   pregnancy and, 203–204
   stress as trigger for, 30–31
Flaxseed oil, 115
Food allergies, 145–146
Foods to avoid, 134–135
Foods to focus on, 132–134. *See also*
   Diet
Forshaw, Joanne, 112
Fox, Katherine, 183–184, 186
Frankincense, 109, 110
Friends' Health Connection, 229, 230
Furtado, Jill, 36

G

Gamma-linoleic acid (GLA), 115–116
Gaspari, Dr. Anthony, 91, 95, 96
Genetics, 31–32, 237
Ginger, 109, 110, 114
Ginkgo, 110, 114
Gold, 93
Government support for lupus research, 234–235
Gross, Dr. Michael, 48, 49–51
Grusd, Dr. Helen, 161, 162, 163

H

Hahnemann, Dr. Samuel, 123
Hair loss
　as lupus symptom, 11, 13, 14, 16, 26
　pregnancy and, 204
　steroids and, 77, 228
　treatment for, 72, 91–92, 96
Hargraves, Dr. Malcolm, 10
Hayden, Robert, 103, 105, 106
Hazlewood, Dr. Carlton F., 127
Headaches, 25–26
Hench, Dr. Phillip, 10
Herbal medicine
　acupuncture and, 106, 108
　drug interactions and, 108, 113, 114
　four herbs for lupus, 109–110
　as mainstream business, 108–109
　possibly helpful herbs, 110–112
Hess, Dr. Evelyn, 146
High blood pressure (hypertension)
　cardiovascular disease and, 136
　corticosteroids and, 78
　NSAIDs and, 70
　pregnancy and, 202, 206
　salt intake and, 136, 139
Hippocrates, 9, 116
History of lupus, 9–11
Hives, 14, 16
Homeopathy, 123–126
Hormonal imbalance, 62
Hormones as triggers, 30, 34, 199–200
Hydrocortisone, 76

Hydrotherapy, 148
Hypertension. *See* High blood pressure
Hypnosis
　defined, 183
　hypnotherapists, 184–186
　self-hypnosis method, 186–187
　visualizing lupus, 183–184

I

Immune factor, 237–238
Immunosuppressive drugs
　description of, 66, 80–83
　kidney disease and, 80–83, 86–87
　pregnancy and, 204, 205
　skin problems and, 93
Imuran (azathioprine)
　description of, 80, 81, 82, 86
　pregnancy and, 202, 204
　skin problems and, 93
Internet resources
　American College of Rheumatology site, 45, 235
　on clinical trials, 246, 247
　online support groups, 230–231, 232
　reputable, 49, 100
Isoniazid (INH), 3, 56

J

Jackson, Dr. April, 147
Jacobs, Dr. Jennifer, 125
Jobs, changing, 212–213. *See also* Work life
Johnson, Robert Wood, 236
Joint pain or swelling, 11, 12–14. *See also* Arthritis

K

Kaposi, Moriz, 10
Katz, Dr. Robert, 75, 77, 78, 81
Kaufman, Karen, 136–140
Kidney disease
　description of, 20–21
　diet and, 135–136
　drug study on, 88

Kidney disease, *continued*
   flaxseed oil for, 115, 139
   high blood pressure and, 136
   immunosuppressive drugs for, 80–83,
      86–87
   LJP 394 clinical trials on, 243–244
   NSAIDs and, 70–71
   success stories, 86–87
   toxemia and, 206
Kidney tests, 59–60
Kimberly, Dr. Robert P., 250, 251
Klee, Celina, 123
Klemperer, Dr. Paul, 10
Klippel, Dr. John H., 20, 21
Koop, C. Everett, 222
Koop's Community, Dr., 232
Kuralt, Charles, 36
Kurtzman, Dr. Neil, 81, 83, 88

L

Laboratory tests
   antibody tests, 60
   anti-DNA antibody test, 57
   antinuclear antibody test (ANA), 41,
      42, 54, 55–57
   anti-Sm antibody test, 58
   blood complement level test, 55, 58
   commonly used, 55
   complete blood count (CBC), 59
   kidney tests, 59–60
   results of, 61
   tissue biopsy, 55, 58
Lactose intolerance, 145
Lahita, Dr. Robert, 88, 145, 155, 160
Lawrence, Dr. Jimmy, 37, 71, 79
Linnik, Dr. Matthew, 243, 244
Lipstick, 33
LJP 394, 243–244
Lockshin, Dr. Michael D., 1, 203, 204,
      205, 206
Lorig, Kate, 226, 227
Lupus. *See also* Diagnosis; Medical
      treatment; Research
   cause of, 5, 236–238
   as complex disease, 1

   depression and, 157–163
   expected course of, 37–38
   four types of, 2–5
   history of, 9–11
   in men, 34–35, 203
   self-test for, 40
   symptoms of, 11–26
   triggers, 26–32
   as a woman's disease, 34
Lupus Awareness Month, 245
Lupus Book, The, 27, 62, 110
Lupus Foundation of America (LFA), 1,
      4, 5, 11, 32, 38, 45, 49, 50, 99,
      100, 227, 235–236, 245
Lupus nephritis. *See also* Kidney disease
   Cytoxan (cyclophosphamide) for,
      81–82, 86, 87
   defined, 20-21
   drug study, 88
   LJP 394 clinical trials on, 243–244
   NSAIDs and, 70–71
   pregnancy and, 202, 206
Lupus Research & Care Amendment of
      2000, 234
LupusLine, 222, 223

M

Madara, Edward, 223, 224, 230, 231
Magnet therapy, 126–128
Malaise or fatigue, 11, 12, 16–17
Marcus, Dr. LindaSusan, 15
Massage
   aromatherapy and, 181–182
   benefits of, 120
   Mary-Jo's story, 116–118
   potential risks of, 121
   types of, 118–119
Massage therapists, 120–121
McDonough, Mary, 5–9, 28
Mease, Philip, 89
Medical treatment. *See also*
      Complementary and alternative
      medicine (CAM)
   DHEA as possible new drug, 85,
      88–90

individualized, 65
for skin problems, 90–97
standard medications, 66–87
Medications as triggers, 29–30, 237
Medications for treatment
antimalarial drugs, 66, 71–74
DHEA and, 85, 88–90
generic and trade names, 67
immunosuppressive drugs, 66, 80–83
nonsteroidal anti-inflammatory drugs
(NSAIDs), 66, 67–71
of skin problems, 90–95
steroids, 66, 75–80
success stories, 86–87
trial-and-error approach to, 83–86
Meek, Carrie, 235
Men with lupus, 34–35, 203
Mental imagery, 175–176
Methotrexate (Immunex)
description of, 80, 82, 84, 85
pregnancy and, 205
for skin problems, 93
Methylprednisolone (Medrol), 76,
77, 204
Mind-body relationship
cognitive-behavioral therapy,
164–170
depression, 157–163
power of the mind, 164
relaxation exercises, 173, 174–187
stress, 30–31, 171–174, 187–188
Misdiagnosis
Eugene's story, 42–44
Gloria Spadaro's story, 45–48
Mary McDonough's story, 5–9, 28
Muscle pain, 18–19
Mustargen (nitrogen mustard), 82
Myers, Mary-Jo, 116–118

N

National Institute of Arthritis and
Musculoskeletal and Skin Diseases
(NIAMS), 235
National Institutes of Health (NIH),
49, 100, 104, 242, 248

National Lupus Alert Day, 245
National Organization for Social
Security Claimant Representatives
(NOSSCR), 221
Neonatal lupus, 4–5, 35–36, 207
Nervous system involvement, 24–26
Nitrogen mustard (Mustargen), 82
Nixon, Richard, 104
Nonsteroidal anti-inflammatory drugs
(NSAIDs)
acupuncture and, 106
alcohol and, 146
for cardiopulmonary complications,
22–23
depression and, 161
description of, 66, 67, 69
generic and trade names of, 68
ideal, 251
side effects of, 69–71
Nutrition
cardiovascular disease and, 136
drug side effects and, 140–142
food allergies, 145–146
foods to avoid, 134–135
foods to focus on, 132–134
guidelines for eating well, 131–132
hunger caused by steroids, 142–145
Karen Kaufman's story, 136–140
kidney disease and, 135–136
vegetarian diet, 134, 138
Nutritional supplements, 114–116, 139

O

O'Connor, Flannery, 36
Oppenheim, Dr. Stefanie, 128
Orasone. *See* Prednisone
Organ-threatening disease
defined, 3
immunosuppressive drugs for, 80–83
remission and, 37
Osler, Sir William, 10
Osteoporosis
Aslera and bone density, 89
calcium supplements for, 85,
140–141

Osteoporosis, *continued*
    diet and, 140–141
    steroids and, 78–79, 84

P

Paknad, Deidre, 213–216
Palmer, David Daniel, 121
Peptide vaccination research, 239
Phillips, Dr. Robert H., 154, 160
Pisetsky, Dr. David S., 238
Plaquenil (hydroxychloroquine
    sulfate)
    description of, 72–73
    eye exams and, 74, 136, 209
    pregnancy and, 204
    side effects of, 74, 84
    for skin problems, 93
Pleurisy, 11, 22, 40
Pneumonitis, 22–23
Prednisolone, 76, 204
Prednisone
    bone scans and, 209
    cholesterol levels and, 142
    defined, 75–76
    Eugene's story, 43
    pregnancy and, 204, 205
    side effects of, 84, 85
    for skin problems, 93
Pregnancy
    acupuncture and, 106
    complications during, 205–206
    flares during, 203–204
    getting pregnant, 200–201
    high-risk, 202
    low-risk, 201
    medications during, 204–205
    questions frequently asked,
      206–208
Progressive muscle relaxation,
    176–177
Pronestyl (procainamide), 3, 56
Protein intake, 134–135
Provost, Dr. Thomas T., 14
Pulse therapy, 76–77

R

Race, 33, 233
Randolph, Pat, 102
Range of motion exercises, 148,
    150–151
Rashes, skin, 11, 12, 14–16, 53
Raynaud's phenomenon
    flaxseed oil for, 115
    gamma-linoleic acid (GLA)
      for, 116
    as lupus symptom, 11, 16
    treating, 64, 209
    in undifferentiated connective tissue
      disease (UCTD), 63
Relaxation
    aromatherapy, 178–182
    benefits of, 173
    biofeedback, 182
    deep breathing, 174–175
    hypnosis, 183–187
    mental imagery, 175–176
    progressive muscle relaxation,
      176–177
Remissions, 18, 37–38
Research
    basic, 238–239
    clinical trials, 238, 241–250
    factors uncovered by, 236–238
    organizations supporting, 234–236
    predictions based on, 250–252
    translational, 238, 239–241
Reston, James, 104
Retinoids, 93
Rheumatoid arthritis
    aerobic exercise for, 152
    ANA test result for, 56
    antimalarial drugs for, 71–72
    as autoimmune disease, 6
    cortisone for, 10
    distinguishing lupus from, 41, 53, 60,
      62, 63
    fish oils for, 114
    gold and, 93
    herbs for, 109, 110

lupus arthritis versus, 14
methotrexate and, 82
Rheumatoid factor (RF) antibody
test, 60
Rodis, Dr. Katina, 165–167, 169
Rogerius, 9
Rogers, Dr. Malcolm P., 36

S

St. John's wort, 110
Salt, 135, 136, 139, 143
Samuelson, Darnell, 89
Scams, 111
Schur, Dr. Peter H., 147
Schwartz, Dr. Robert S., 17, 19
Seal, 36
Second opinions, 51
Selenium, 133–134
Self-reactive B cell research, 239
Self-test for lupus, 40
Serra, Father Junipero, 37, 38
Sex, 198–200
Sex hormones
estrogen, 30, 34, 89, 199
lupus and, 88–89
Shapiro, Dr. Howard S., 159,
160, 162
Sherer, Dr. Renslow, 116
Singh, R.R., 239
Sjögren's syndrome
as lupus-like disorder, 56, 63–64
sex and, 198
symptoms of, 63, 209
Skin problems
evolving therapies for, 91, 94–95
rashes, 11, 12, 14–16, 53
steroids and, 77–78
sun tips for, 94
surgical treatments for, 91,
95–97
systemic therapy for, 90, 92–93
topical treatment for, 90, 91–92
Smith, Dr. D. Edwards, 113

Social Security disability (SSD)
benefits
filing for, 218–221
Orlando's story, 216–218
Sohmer, Alec G., 219, 220, 221
Spadaro, Gloria, 45–48
Spiegel, Dr. David, 225
Statistical facts, 34
Stem cell transplantation, 244–245
Steroids
children and, 79
cholesterol levels and, 142
depression and, 161
description of, 75–77
hunger caused by, 142–145
pregnancy and, 204
side effects of, 77–80, 161
Stevens, Dr. Mary Betty, 13
Stohl, Dr. William, 240
Stone, Al, 105
Strength training exercises, 148, 150,
153–154
Stress
avoiding, 187–188
effects of, 30–31, 171–174
as environmental factor, 237
relaxation to counteract, 173,
174–187
Stretching exercises, 150, 151–152
Sulfa-based drugs, 3, 29–30
Sun tips, 94
Sunlight (ultraviolet light)
blocking UV rays, 91, 92, 94
as environmental factor, 237
as lupus trigger, 28, 29
photosensitivity, 53
Sun-protected clothing, 92
Sunscreen, 91, 94
Support groups
benefits of, 221–222, 224–226
finding a group, 222–224
online, 230–231, 232
problems in, 226–227
Symptom diary, 102, 103

Symptoms
    blood disorders, 19–20
    cardiopulmonary complications,
        22–23
    common, 11, 12–26
    fever, 17, 18
    hair loss, 14, 16, 26, 228
    joint pain or swelling, 11, 12–14
    kidney disease, 20–21
    malaise or fatigue, 11, 16–17
    muscle pain, 18–19
    nervous system involvement, 24–26
    skin rash, 11, 12, 14–16
    talking about, 192–193
    variability in, 12
Syphilis test results, 52, 54
Systemic lupus erythematosus (SLE).
        See also Lupus
    blood disorders and, 19–20
    in children, 36–37
    defined, 2–3
    expected course of, 37–38
    fatigue and, 16–17
    joint pain or swelling and, 11, 12–14
    nervous system involvement in, 24–26
    skin lesions, 14, 15

T

Tests. *See* Laboratory tests
Thalidomide, 95
Thompson, Margrey, 148–153, 155, 209
Thrombocytopenia, 19, 77
Tissue biopsy, 55, 58
Toxemia, 204, 206
Translational research, 238, 239–241
Traynor, Dr. Ann, 244, 245
Treatment. *See* Complementary and
        alternative medicine (CAM);
        Medications for treatment
Triggers
    chemical factors, 27–28, 29
    common, 29
    defined, 26–27
    genetics, 29, 31–32, 237

    medications, 29–30, 237
    stress, 29, 30–31, 237
    ultraviolet light, 28, 29, 53, 94, 237
Turmeric, 109, 110

U

Ultraviolet light
    blocking UV rays, 91, 92, 94
    as environmental factor, 237
    as lupus trigger, 28, 29
    photosensitivity, 53
Undifferentiated connective tissue
        disease (UCTD), 62–63
Upledger, Dr. John E., 123

V

Vaccinations, 81
Vallbona, Dr. Carlos, 127, 128
van Vollenhoven, Dr. Ronald, 90
Vegetarian diet, 134, 138
Veritas Medicine Web site, 246
Vitamin D, 140–141
Vitamin E, 133
von Hebra, Ferdinand, 10

W

Wallace, Dr. Daniel J., 2, 4, 12, 24, 27,
        37, 38, 62–63, 73, 79, 199, 200,
        251, 252
Walport, Mark, 241
Warner, Charles Dudley, 226
Water exercise classes, 148
Water therapy, 180–181
Weinstein, Dr. Arthur, 69
White blood cell counts, 20, 54, 59
Willan, Dr., 9
Women
    African American, 33
    breast implants, 6–7, 8, 28
    lipstick, 33
    lupus in, 34
    oral contraceptives, 30, 199–200
    pregnancy, 200–208
    sick mom's story, 208–210

Wong, Dr. George, 111, 112
Work life
    changing jobs, 212–213
    Deidre Paknad's story, 213–216
    finding balance, 211–212
    telling boss/coworkers, 210–211

Y

Yee, Dr. John, 241, 242, 249, 250
Young, Gwendolyn, 211–212

Z

Zinc, 114, 134, 135

Improve Your Health and Avoid Problems When Using Common Medications and Natural Supplements Together

Millions of people, just like you, use vitamins or herbs along with prescription and nonprescription medications without knowing that some combinations are beneficial while some can be downright dangerous.

Based on the revolutionary electronic Internet database *Healthnotes Online*, this book is written by the most trusted and respected experts in natural medicine who have created the only natural health information resource that is both comprehensive and user-friendly.

The *A–Z Guide to Drug-Herb-Vitamin Interactions 2nd edition* helps you learn which drugs can deplete your body's essential nutrients; which supplements can help your prescriptions work better, or reduce drug side effects; and which herbs and drugs should never be taken together.

healthnotes®

The #1 Name in Natural Health Information

A–Z Guide to Drug-Herb-Vitamin Interactions

Revised and Expanded 2nd Edition

Improve Your Health and Avoid Side Effects
When Using Common Medications
and Natural Supplements Together

EDITED BY ALAN R. GABY, M.D.,
AND THE HEALTHNOTES MEDICAL TEAM

Covers more than 18,000 interactions!

ISBN 978-0-307-33664-4 / Paperback
464 pages / U.S. $22.95 / Can. $32.95

THREE
RIVERS
PRESS

Available everywhere books are sold.
Visit us online at www.crownpublishing.com.

Rejuvenate and Refresh Your Body Starting Today

There is an effective way to free yourself of chronic aches and pain, feel healthier, and be more energetic. It's called *detoxification,* a process that stimulates your body's natural ability to cleanse itself. Inside, you'll discover a simple seven-day detoxification program that will help you improve resistance to disease, normalize weight, and increase physical and mental stamina. Completely updated and revised, this edition features:

- Easy-to-prepare recipes
- Sample menu plans
- And everything else you need to begin your new life of healthier living—today!

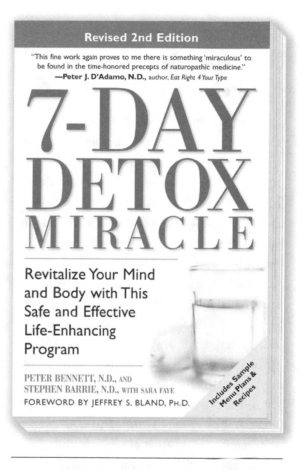

ISBN 978-0-7516-3097-8/ Paperback
400 pages / U.S. $16.95 / Can. $25.95

THREE RIVERS PRESS

Available everywhere books are sold.
Visit us online at www.crownpublishing.com.

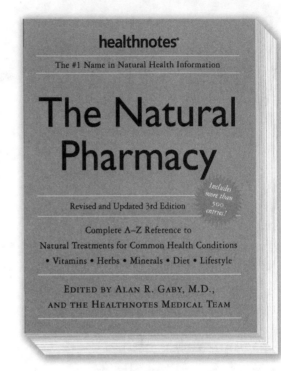

About the Author

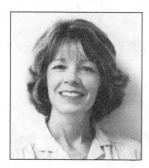

Theresa Foy DiGeronimo, M.Ed., is the author of numerous health books, including *New Hope for People with Fibromyalgia*, and is coauthor of *Living Foods for Optimum Health*. An adjunct professor teaching undergraduate and graduate writing courses at the William Paterson University of New Jersey, she lives in Hawthorne, New Jersey.

About the Medical Reviewer

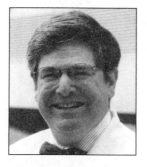

Stephen A. Paget, M.D., FACR, FACP, is the chairman of the Division of Rheumatology, Physician-in-Chief, and member of the over-sight board of the Kirkland Center for Lupus Research at Hospital for Special Surgery. He is also the Joseph P. Routh Professor of Medicine at the Weill Medical College of Cornell University and an attending physician at the New York Presbyterian Hospital. He is currently the President of the New York Rheumatism Association as well as a member of the Board of Trustees at the New York chapter of the Arthritis Foundation and the Board of Governors of the Burke Rehabilitation Center. Dr. Paget serves on other committees in various institutions nationwide. He lives with his family in New York City.